BUILDING SOUND BONES AND MUSCLES

TIME
LIFE ®
BOOKS

Other Publications:

PLANET EARTH
COLLECTOR'S LIBRARY OF THE CIVIL WAR
CLASSICS OF THE OLD WEST
THE EPIC OF FLIGHT
THE GOOD COOK
THE SEAFARERS
THE ENYCLOPEDIA OF COLLECTIBLES
THE GREAT CITIES
WORLD WAR II
HOME REPAIR AND IMPROVEMENT
THE WORLD'S WILD PLACES
THE TIME-LIFE LIBRARY OF BOATING
HUMAN BEHAVIOR
THE ART OF SEWING
THE OLD WEST
THE EMERGENCE OF MAN
THE AMERICAN WILDERNESS
THE TIME-LIFE ENCYCLOPEDIA OF GARDENING
LIFE LIBRARY OF PHOTOGRAPHY
THIS FABULOUS CENTURY
FOODS OF THE WORLD
TIME-LIFE LIBRARY OF AMERICA
TIME-LIFE LIBRARY OF ART
GREAT AGES OF MAN
LIFE SCIENCE LIBRARY
THE LIFE HISTORY OF THE UNITED STATES
TIME READING PROGRAM
LIFE NATURE LIBRARY
LIFE WORLD LIBRARY

FAMILY LIBRARY:
HOW THINGS WORK IN YOUR HOME
THE TIME-LIFE BOOK OF THE FAMILY CAR
THE TIME-LIFE FAMILY LEGAL GUIDE
THE TIME-LIFE BOOK OF FAMILY FINANCE

*This volume is one of a series designed to familiarize readers
with the latest advances in medical science as a guide in
maintaining their own health and fitness.*

BUILDING SOUND **BONES AND MUSCLES**

by Oliver E. Allen

AND THE EDITORS OF TIME-LIFE BOOKS

LIBRARY OF HEALTH / TIME-LIFE BOOKS / ALEXANDRIA, VIRGINIA

THE AUTHOR:
Oliver E. Allen, formerly a Time-Life Books editor and planning director, brought to this work not only his long experience in writing but also unplanned firsthand research on fractures and how they heal: While preparing this volume he fell off a stepladder and broke both his wrists. Given the kind of treatment he describes in Chapter 5, they mended promptly. His previous books include two volumes in The Seafarers series, *The Windjammers* and *The Pacific Navigators,* and, for the Epic of Flight series, *The Airline Builders.*

THE CONSULTANTS:
Dr. Roy C. Swan is the Joseph C. Hinsey Professor of Anatomy at Cornell University Medical College in New York City, where he served as Chairman of the Department of Anatomy from 1959 to 1978. He received his M.D. degree from Cornell in 1947.

For information about any Time-Life book, please write:
Reader Information, Time-Life Books,
541 North Fairbanks Court, Chicago, Illinois 60611.

First printing. Printed in U.S.A.
Published simultaneously in Canada.
School and library distribution by Silver Burdett Company, Morristown, New Jersey.

TIME-LIFE is a trademark of Time Incorporated U.S.A.

Library of Congress Cataloguing in Publication Data
The Editors of Time-Life Books
  Building Sound Bones and Muscles
  (Library of Health)
  Bibliography p.
  Includes index.
  1. Musculoskeletal system.   2. Musculoskeletal
system—Diseases.
  I. Time-Life Books.   II. Series.   III. Title.
  (DNLM: 1. Musculoskeletal system—Popular works.
  WE 100 A428b)
QP301.A35   616.7   81-18208
ISBN 0-8094-3788-0   AACR2
ISBN 0-8094-3787-2 (lib. bdg.)
ISBN 0-8094-3786-4 (retail ed.)

LIBRARY OF HEALTH

Editor: Martin Mann
Editorial Staff for *Building Sound Bones and Muscles*
Senior Editor: William Frankel
Assistant Editor: Phyllis K. Wise
Designer: Albert Sherman
Picture Editor: Jane Speicher Jordan
Text Editors: Laura Longley, C. Tyler Mathisen, Brian McGinn
Writers: Deborah Berger-Turnbull, Jean Getlein, Peter Kaufman, Donia Whiteley Mills
Researchers: Norma E. Kennedy, James Robert Stengel (principals), Judy French, John Ethan Hankins, Erin Taylor Monroney, Fran Moshos, Trudy W. Pearson, Jules Taylor
Assistant Designer: Cynthia T. Richardson
Copy Coordinators: Margery duMond, Stephen G. Hyslop
Picture Coordinator: Rebecca C. Christoffersen
Editorial Assistant: Nana Heinbaugh Juarbe
Special Contributors: Christopher S. Conner, Lydia Preston, Sterling Seagrave, Dr. Edward L. Zimney (writers); Barbara Lerner (researcher)

EDITORIAL OPERATIONS

Production Director: Feliciano Madrid
Assistants: Peter A. Inchauteguiz, Karen A. Meyerson
Copy Processing: Gordon E. Buck
Quality Control Director: Robert L. Young
Assistant: James J. Cox
Associates: Daniel J. McSweeney, Michael G. Wight
Art Coordinator: Anne B. Landry
Copy Room Director: Susan B. Galloway
Assistants: Celia Beattie, Ricki Tarlow

Correspondents: Elisabeth Kraemer (Bonn); Margot Hapgood, Dorothy Bacon (London); Susan Jonas, Lucy T. Voulgaris (New York); Maria Vincenza Aloisi, Josephine du Brusle (Paris); Ann Natanson (Rome). Valuable assistance was also given by: Joanne Reid (Chicago); Judy Aspinall, Christine Hinze, Millicent Trowbridge (London); Carolyn T. Chubet, Diane Cook, Miriam Hsia, Christina Lieberman (New York); Mimi Murphy (Rome); Annelise Schulz (Vienna).

CONTENTS

CHAPTER 1

A curious arrangement for living upright

New ways to fix the frame
A divinely built mansion
Building strength into the structure
The importance of food
Joints for a lifetime of flexibility
Matched muscles for every movement

Imagine a somewhat rubbery, irregularly shaped contraption weighing perhaps 100 to 200 pounds, measuring some five or six feet in length and containing a number of internal sticks and posts, most of which do not touch each other. Such an object would appear to be lumpish and unmanageable. Prop it up on one end, somehow balancing it on the two narrow, flexible protuberances that seem meant as supports, and it turns out to be top-heavy. How can it ever stand up?

Yet it does—for minutes, months, a lifetime. Not only that, it moves. It can perform cartwheels, climb mountains, heft dumbbells, hurl balls at almost 100 miles an hour, pole-vault 18 feet and execute a ballerina's arabesques. It is that most extraordinary contrivance, the human body. Tough, efficient, it owes its power and versatility—as well as its grace—to an intricate, ingeniously connected system of bones and muscles that actually improves with use. A cage held up by elastic bands, the human frame endures as a working monument to the defiance of the laws of physics.

Few things in life bring so much pleasure as a well-functioning frame. By the same token, few things can be as irritating and painful as bones and muscles that have fallen victim to the multifarious ills that can beset them. While accommodating endless intricate movement over the years, bones and muscles absorb an immense amount of wear and tear and even abuse. Poor habits can bring on backaches and foot aches, accidents can strain muscles and break bones, illness can leave joints inflamed and ultimately immobile.

According to authorities at the Yale University School of Medicine, ailments of the frame rank first among disease groups that affect the quality of life. In total economic cost they are second only to diseases of the heart and blood vessels—$20 billion annually is spent on them in the United States. About 20 million Americans are affected by these diseases; in any year one person in 10 can expect to suffer a fracture, dislocation, sprain or strain. A survey in Sweden found that 60 per cent of adult men had endured low-back pain. Furthermore, commented the Yale experts, "arthritis is almost universal in the elderly."

Contemporary life often gets the blame for the troubles people have with their bones and muscles. Certainly the painful whiplash injury, which helps bring more than eight million dollars a year to the makers of braces in the United States, was almost unknown before the invention of the automobile; and the spiral fracture of the tibia, one of the lower leg bones, was similarly rare until downhill skiing became a mass sport after World War II. In addition, labor-saving machinery and sit-down jobs have eliminated exertions that once kept muscles strong and joints limber. The results are sprains, aching backs, inflammation and stiffness.

But a major fault lies in the magnificent frame itself and is an unfortunate by-product of evolution. The epochal move by some human ancestor several million years ago, in which he swung out of the trees and began walking not on all fours but erect, the torso vertical instead of horizontal, conferred on him certain unique advantages. Standing tall, these early humans could see farther and move faster, and their hands

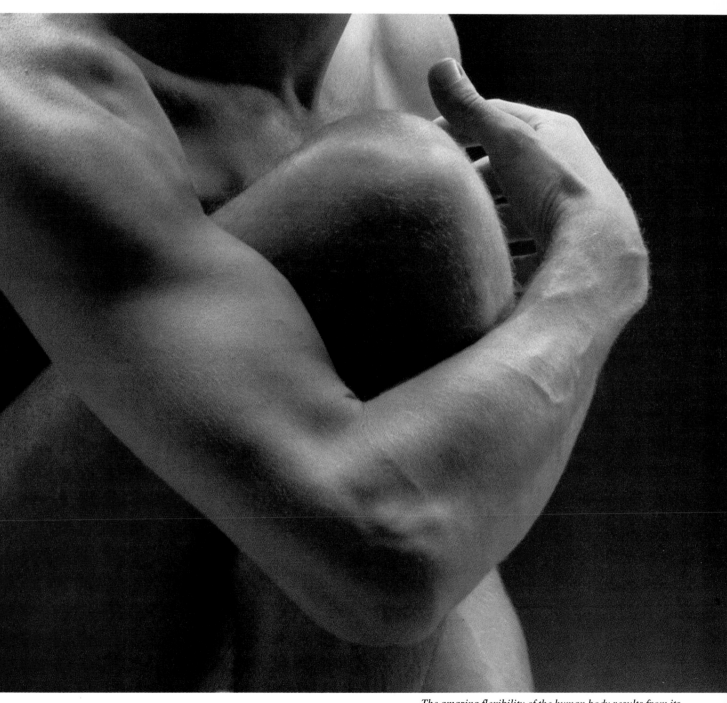

The amazing flexibility of the human body results from its elaborate system of bones, muscles, connective tissues and movable joints. The joints require the most care—they bear the brunt of life's wear and tear—and particularly in the arms, legs and hands they make possible the peculiarly human motions of upright walking and dextrous manipulation.

were freed for actions that swiftly brought them superiority over all other creatures. No other mammal is truly erect as humans are—not even apes, who now and then return to all fours, and who cannot walk backward. The body these human ancestors bequeathed to their descendants is still adapting to the new attitude. When humans began walking on their hind legs, they set up the causes of backache.

A knee repaired in one day

There is nothing much anyone can do about evolution. But there is a great deal everyone can do about backaches and most of the other ills of the paradoxically sturdy yet frail human frame. New drugs and surgical techniques repair much damage that once caused prolonged suffering: The delicate job of removing torn cartilage from the knee, which once required one or two weeks in the hospital, is now performed with a device that lets the surgeon work inside the knee without cutting it open. Some patients can go home, walking on the repaired knee, the same day.

Effective treatments now exist for many deformities, present at birth, that once ruined lives. Clubfoot, a common birth defect in which the foot and leg turn inward, can now be corrected in 60 per cent of the cases by simple measures: plaster casts, braces and special shoes that are needed only two years. For the other 40 per cent, surgery to straighten certain bones or to lengthen the tendon from the leg to the heel corrects the condition. The old remedy for arthritis— gold—is still favored, but new drugs such as cortisone, phenylbutazone, carisoprodol and ibuprofen often bring quick recovery or relief from sprains, bruises and the swollen joints of bursitis. Even the ancient art of setting broken bones, practiced successfully since prehistoric times, has been revolutionized by the invention of metal pins to hold the pieces of a broken bone together until they mend.

The radical change made by newer treatment is illustrated by the case of a 23-year-old man who recently broke his femur—the body's largest and strongest bone, connecting the hip to the knee—in a motorcycle accident. Before World War II such a break would have had him out of action for the better part of a year—immobilized in bed for six to nine months in a cast that encased him from chest to toes, and forced to use crutches six to 10 weeks thereafter.

Instead, three pins—thin, springy steel bars 18 inches long—were inserted in the femur to support his weight while the break mended. After the surgeon realigned the two pieces of broken bone, he made small incisions on either side of the leg just above the knee, and drilled half-inch holes into the bone. Then he twisted the flexible pins into the holes and up through the hollow center of the bone until the pins emerged from the bone and their ends splayed outward, securely locking the halves of the broken bone into a solid unit.

Within a week the young man was up and about on crutches; after a month he needed only a cane, and he discarded that within three months. Six months after the accident the two outer pins were removed in a second operation. By the time a year had passed, the patient was jogging 14 miles a week—one pin was still in place, but was ready to be removed, leaving him with a leg almost as good as new.

Perhaps as important as advanced treatment is the growing understanding of ways to prevent injuries—even those that seem unavoidable. Exercise offers one way. It strengthens muscles—weak abdominal muscles, for example, are a main cause of back injury. In addition, the pulling of active muscles on bones makes bones grow larger and stronger. And exercise lets the body reach its potential for action. The virtuoso escape artist Harry Houdini, who sometimes seemed to make his hands smaller than his wrists, credited many of his feats to exercise. Every muscle in his body—in his shoulders, arms, wrists, torso, thighs, ankles—was ready to do his bidding, and should his dextrous fingers be tied up, his toes opened the padlocks that bound him.

Sir William Arbuthnot Lane, a Scottish bone specialist of the 19th Century, said that he could tell from a man's bones how he earned his living: Different work—shoveling coal, making shoes or driving a brewery wagon—stressed different sets of muscles and stimulated particular bones to grow larger and stronger. More recently, a study on the effect of athletic activity on bone development compared X-rays of the hands and forearms of expert tennis players with those of people who did not play tennis; the comparison showed that the tennis players had longer forearm bones in the racket arm.

Conversely, bones, like muscles, will start to atrophy or waste away in periods of idleness. Some of the early astronauts lost as much as 20 per cent of their bone content while living in a weightless environment without exercise. (They quickly regained it upon their return.)

Protection against injury may also be afforded by the right equipment. It can forestall many injuries not only in sports but in everyday activities; whiplash would once again be rare if all drivers adjusted their seat headrests to skull height. Correctly fitted shoes can eliminate aches all over the body.

Most of all, knowing how to use the body structure protects it from harm. Expert skiers do not break legs nearly so often as overconfident duffers. Certain methods of sitting, standing, carrying and lifting block fatigue and injury.

Protecting an ''exquisite structure''

These ways of sustaining the extraordinary power and versatility of the human frame rest on knowledge of its construction. ''It seems to me highly dishonourable for a Reasonable Soul to live in so Divinely built a Mansion,'' observed 17th Century English physicist Robert Boyle, ''altogether unacquainted with the exquisite Structure of it.'' Acquaintanceship with that exquisite structure can help the reasonable soul within it to avoid situations that lead to trouble—and to recognize problems that do occur for what they are.

That people initiated this acquaintanceship long ago is evident in carvings on walls of prehistoric caves and in hieroglyphics in Egyptian tombs, but until Claudius Galen, born in 130 A.D. in the Greek city of Pergamum, studied the anatomy of humans and animals, knowledge of the subject remained sketchy at best.

The son of an architect, Galen studied medicine in Alexandria, the leading medical center of the Roman Empire, and by the age of 28 he was back practicing in his hometown as doctor to the gladiators, a job that gave him ample opportunity to observe bones and muscles in action. But Galen was hampered in his anatomical studies—as were a number of important anatomists to follow him—by the difficulty of obtaining human cadavers for dissection, a problem he dis-

cussed in detail in his treatise ''On Anatomical Procedure'':

''The human bones are subjects of study with which you should first become perfectly familiar,'' he counseled students. ''At Alexandria this is very easy, since the physicians in that country accompany the instruction they give to their students with opportunities for personal inspection during autopsies. Hence you must try to get to Alexandria for this reason alone, if for no other. But if you cannot manage this, still it is not impossible to obtain a view of human bones. Personally I have very often had a chance to do this where tombs or monuments have become broken up.

''On one occasion a river, having risen to the level of a grave that had been carelessly constructed a few months previously, easily disintegrated it,'' Galen continued. ''The water carried the corpse downstream for the distance of a league, and coming to a lake-like stretch with sloping banks, deposited it. There it lay ready for inspection, just as though prepared by a doctor for his pupil's lesson.''

Because Galen had such difficulty in acquiring human

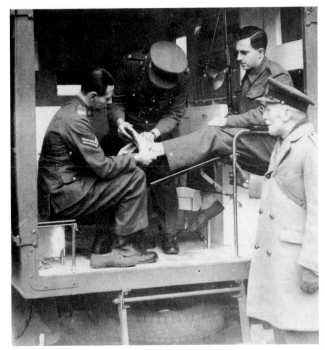

Seated in World War II's first mobile chiropody unit—a van stocked with foot-care supplies and instruments—a British soldier has his aching arches examined by a medical officer (center), by the unit's operator (left), and by a curious bystander. Beginning in 1941, this lorry aided troops who suffered corns, calluses and ''march fractures''—bone cracks caused by constant walking.

cadavers for study, he frequently turned to apes and other animals—a recourse that led him to inaccurate observations about human anatomy. He endowed all human beings, for instance, with a seven-segmented breastbone and, like later literal interpreters of the Bible, he gave man one less rib than woman. Yet Galen's observations, recorded by him in textbooks, were considered definitive in the West for more than a thousand years. Physicians in Asia acquired more accurate information; the famous 10th Century fable of The Thousand and One Arabian Nights, for example, includes a long passage detailing with great accuracy the bones of the human frame, from the skull right down to the big toe.

Not until the early 16th Century did such knowledge become available to European physicians. The great Italian artist Leonardo da Vinci picked up where Galen left off, dissecting more than 30 cadavers while in the service of the Borgia family and producing more than a thousand drawings of human anatomy, detailing not only the bones but the muscular system and the actions of each muscle. But his extraordinary notebooks were not found for two centuries, and the modern explanation of human anatomy began with the work of the Brussels physician Andreas Vesalius. Like Galen, he had trouble getting cadavers for dissection—he cut down from gibbets the bodies of hanged criminals.

Over the years since Vesalius published his observations in seven major books—one of which gave Adam back his missing rib—the paradoxical uniformity and variability of the human frame has become clear. Its size and shape are extremely variable: The Masai of Africa have very long thin bones that make some of the men seven feet tall; Eskimos have shorter bones that give them an average height of about five feet five. Gender makes a difference. Women's bones and muscles are generally smaller than men's, and certain critical parts, such as the hip and sacrum bones of the pelvis, are easily distinguishable as male or female.

But the total number of bones is constant. Babies are born with some 350 bones, all of them "soft"—composed mostly of a watery substance called cartilage. In the process of growth the cartilage is calcified—stiffened by the addition of a great deal of the mineral calcium phosphate. Then most particles of the calcified cartilage are replaced by true bone, which is largely calcium phosphate, and some of the 350 separate pieces fuse. The normal adult grows up with between 206 and 209 bones—the possible extras found in some healthy people include one or two additional ribs near the neck and another bone in the coccyx, or tailbone.

These bones form the intricate scaffolding that gives *Homo sapiens* not only his familiar shape but the support and protection he needs as well. Almost every one of the bones does double or even triple duty. The core of the entire system, the spinal column, is an intricate assemblage of 26 oddly shaped flattish bones, called vertebrae, that are separated by cushioning tissue called discs. The spine not only holds up the head and trunk while permitting them to turn and bend but tightly clasps the vital central nerve cord. Above this backbone the skull surrounds the brain with a solid layer of armor, shields the eyes and other sensory organs, and comes equipped with a large movable part—the jaw.

Branching out from the spine are 12 (or 13) pairs of ribs, which support and protect the heart and lungs, and move slightly with every breath, 14 to 20 times a minute for a lifetime. The bones of the shoulder-girdle at the top of the trunk and those of the pelvis at the bottom loosely anchor the limbs and, by means of ingenious joints, permit a range of movements gymnasts and dancers vie to demonstrate.

The limbs themselves—each with its single big upper bone, two lower bones, complex wrist or ankle and five supple digits—have myriad uses: The legs support and move this flexible frame while the arms perform endless tasks and sometimes extraordinary feats. "A cat climbs, an antelope leaps, a chamois scales mountains," observed one admirer of human capability. "Man, without their special physical equipment, accomplishes all these feats and many more besides that only he has thought of."

Escaping the troubles of walking upright

Admirable as it is, the hard-working skeleton is in some ways a less-than-ideal structure. For one thing, its upright stance leaves the midsection vulnerable: While the brain, heart and lungs are thoroughly shielded, the pelvis does an inadequate

Conditioning bodies for strength and grace

For professional ballet dancers, leg injuries, back pain and such foot ailments as bunions and calluses are occupational hazards of a career that has been rated second only to professional football for the intensity of its demands on the body. Ballet dancers know that the best defense against such maladies is a good offense. Throughout their schooling and careers, dancers exercise rigorously and religiously, conditioning their bodies to withstand the stresses of their profession.

Although ballet exercises are of necessity specialized and strenuous, many of them are similar to those that are helpful to ordinary people who want to attain similar goals of flexibility and strength. What is more, dancers, like other active people, recognize that exercises offer more than physical benefits: They can condition the mind as well as the body. The connection between physical prowess and mental agility was suggested by ballet superstar Mikhail Baryshnikov. Once asked which part of his body he worries about most, Baryshnikov said nothing. He simply pointed to his head.

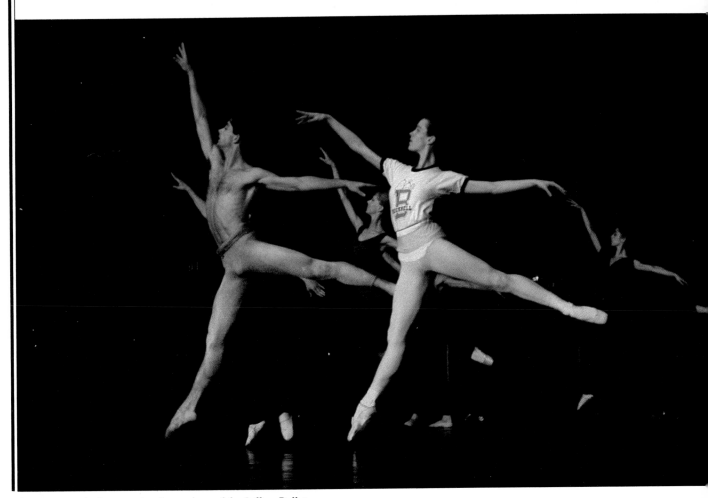

Arms outstretched, toes pointed, members of the Joffrey Ballet rehearse a graceful arabesque leap at Wolf Trap Farm Park, Virginia. The dancers' ability to perform this delicate yet demanding maneuver —and to do so with little fear of injury —is predicated on extensive, regular exercise.

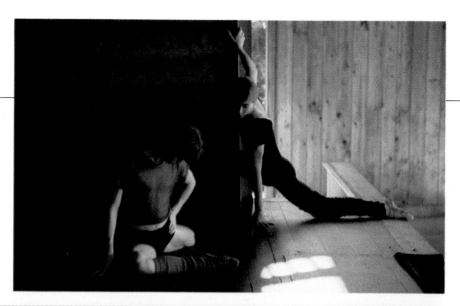

Two dancers execute warm-up exercises
that, like any well-conceived routine, stretch
their muscles gently at first, then harder.
The seated dancer twists his trunk easily in a
maneuver that loosens the muscles of his
hips and groin. His partner, arms positioned
for balance, squats on legs thrust
forward and back, stretching the hamstring
muscles on the back of his right leg and
the muscles of his groin.

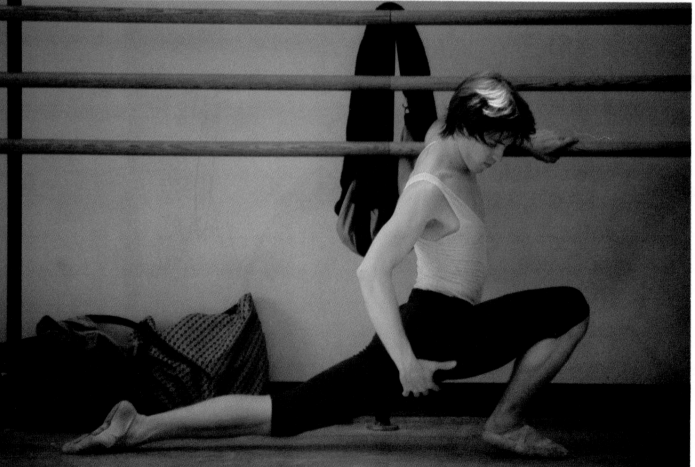

At the barre, a student at the School of American Ballet lunges
onto his right leg while extending his left. The exercise flexes the
muscles on the upper rear of his right leg, including the gluteus
maximus and the hamstring, as well as the quadriceps on the front
of his left thigh. By adopting a similar position—but not
lunging—nondancers can toughen their own leg muscles.

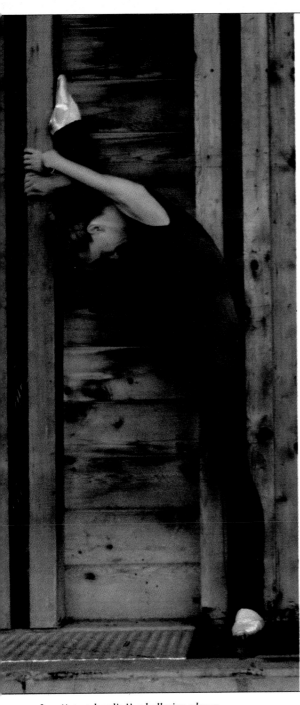

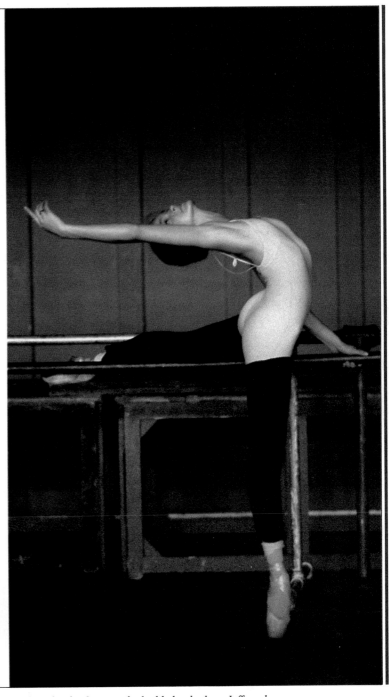

In a "stretch split," a ballerina places her right leg above her head against a wall while she pulls her shoulders forward. The move stretches the hamstring and other muscles on her right leg, and also the muscles of her shoulder.

Arching her back to nearly double her body, a Joffrey dancer stretches virtually every muscle along the front of her body, from her neck to the toes of her right foot. The exercise promotes whole-body flexibility in a single motion, but a series of less complex actions can produce similar effects: Rolling the head slowly in circles, for example, can loosen neck muscles.

job of guarding the abdomen. Through the eons the pelvis has become much wider to allow for the extra weight it must bear—wider in women than in men, to facilitate childbearing—but it provides protection and control only at the back and at the sides. The front is ungirdled.

If human beings still walked on all fours, the thighs would help shield the abdomen, which would hang in simple fashion from the generally horizontal spine, its weight distributed evenly. The digestive organs would rest gently on the abdominal floor. All of that has changed since the structure was tipped on end. The floor has become a more-or-less vertical wall, and the abdomen is hardly supported except by muscles—which tend to weaken in their fight against gravity's downward pull. The strain is compounded by obesity, for extra fat tends to collect on the abdomen, adding to the load that the stomach muscles—and the spine—must support.

The spine itself has undergone significant changes because of mankind's two-legged stance. Whereas in four-legged creatures the spine is called upon to do little more than enclose the spinal nerve cord and link up the ribs, pelvis and limbs, in humans the added chore of supporting most of the body's weight has made it a heavily burdened vertical pole, subject to all sorts of compression and twisting forces.

To handle this assignment, the spine has taken on a couple of curves in addition to the one or two it presented when it was horizontal, until now it has a kind of double-S shape. At the base of the neck the spine curves outward around the shoulder-blade region, to support the ribs. Approaching the lower back it goes back in, then out again. Finally, after joining with the pelvis, it takes a last curve inward, ending between the hips in the coccyx—a vestigial tail. All those curves give the spine great flexibility, permitting easy bending and also protecting the body against sudden shocks such as those incurred in leaping off a bus. If one of the curves is accentuated through faulty posture or some other cause, or if the spinal column is subjected to undue strain, the delicate arrangement of bones can be upset, often painfully.

When the legs began to bear all the body's weight instead of sharing the burden with the other two limbs, their bones too were altered somewhat. The upper end of the thighbone,

which makes a turn so that its head can fit securely into the pelvis while still retaining an impressive range of motion, became thicker and thus more resistant to injury. At the opposite end of the leg, the foot was called upon not just to place a single point on the ground for balance—most four-footed mammals walk on their toes—but to provide stability. So the heel, which in other creatures is a modest appendage not even touching the ground, has become quite large, assisting the human balancing act, and the foot has developed a series of arches—because an arch provides much greater strength than a flat form and this structural shape makes the foot an admirable weight-bearer.

Through evolution, therefore, the entire human frame and its individual bones became extremely strong but at the same time remarkably resilient. Although the skeleton's total weight comes to little more than 20 pounds, it is capable of bearing incredible loads. Olympic champion Vasily Alexeev of the U.S.S.R. once lifted 562.7 pounds of steel barbells. The Cristiani family, circus acrobats who began thrilling audiences across Europe and America in the late 19th Century, perfected the human column—four men balancing on one another's shoulders in testimony to the body's strength and muscle control. First one, then another, then a third vaulted off a board, spinning up and arriving atop the previous vaulter's shoulders. The low man on this column shouldered a combined weight of more than 400 pounds.

Tests on the laboratory machines used to measure the strength of metal bars have proved that bones from cadavers can take even more weight than is indicated by the Cristiani brothers' performance. A shinbone could hold up an automobile containing four passengers. Yet if bone were not as flexible as it is strong—if it were more like metal—it would break far more readily than it does. Almost 20 times more resilient than steel, bone is as flexible as it is strong because of the way it is made and what it is made of.

How bones are made strong

That bones are as strong as they are is particularly remarkable in view of the fact that they start out in the soft form of cartilage. The semi-finished state is all-important when a baby is being delivered from the mother's womb—the infant skull, formed of several separate and flexible plates, can be compressed slightly as it passes through the narrow birth canal, and other bones are pliable enough to follow effortlessly. Soon after the first breath, the baby's skull starts to knit together; during the first year a gap at the apex remains, evidence that the process is not yet fully completed. Other bones begin to harden, too, as calcium phosphate from foods is deposited in the hardening, growing bones in two forms. Solid, compact material, covered by a membrane called the periosteum, makes up the outer shell of the familiar hard cylinder. So-called cancellous bone—spongelike, porous material—honeycombs the cylinders' interior, particularly the knobby ends of the longer bones.

Filling the spaces in the cancellous bone—and, by a roundabout route, helping to build all bone—is a soft substance called marrow, manufacturing site for the white blood cells that fight disease in the body and the red blood cells that carry oxygen throughout the whole system. The marrow is tunneled by vessels that take freshly made red and white cells out and also bring in red cells laden with nutrients the bone needs for life and growth. "With the help of blood," wrote the noted writer on natural history, John Stewart Collis, "we build bones, and within bones thus made by blood we create more blood to make more bones."

It was long thought that after bone replaced cartilage, the bones grew from the inside out. But in the 18th Century Henri-Louis Duhamel, a French country squire who, like many well-to-do contemporaries, dabbled in scientific experimentation, challenged this idea. He fed his chickens, pigs, turkeys and pigeons food colored with a red dye called madder, which had been found to turn bones red. Duhamel discovered upon cutting a bone crosswise that the inner bone was white and only the outer layer red. Because the red layer had to come from the most recently eaten food, the outermost layer was the newest one.

Later that century the Scotsman John Hunter, who had begun his adult life as an apprentice to a cabinetmaker and then joined his anatomist brother as an assistant, took up the madder experiments. He alternated feedings on his animals

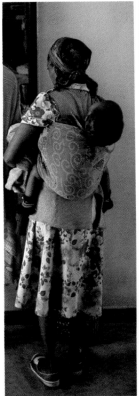
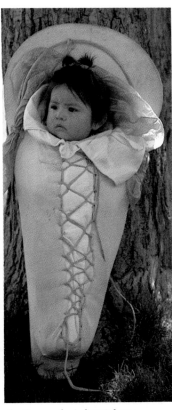

Babies who are swaddled like the Comanche infant (above right) are much more likely to suffer dislocated hips in later life than are babies carried in a back-sling like the one used by the Kenyan mother at left. The sling keeps legs naturally flexed and turned outward; swaddling rigidly extends the legs in an abnormal position that aggravates the congenital hip-joint weakness common among infants, sometimes causing the thighbone to pop out of place. Such dislocations are common not only among North American Indians but also among Laplanders, who swaddle babies as well; the ailment is rare among Eskimos, Chinese and many Africans, who, like the Kenyan mother, carry their infants in slings.

so that the outer, new bone alternated in color, with the dyed or undyed food. He then stopped dyeing the food for several weeks before killing an animal. And he discovered that the innermost red layer disappeared—the older bone near the marrow was somehow absorbed into body tissue. New bone, he concluded, was laid down by the periosteum, the outer shell around already-existing bone.

The mechanism of this creation of new bone and absorption of old gradually became understood following the identification of two types of cells: One type, called osteoblasts, makes bone, and the other, called osteoclasts, destroys bone. Working in a wonderfully cooperative way, the osteoblasts build new bone material on the outside while their much larger companions, the osteoclasts, diligently remove the old, unneeded material on the inside.

In this way, the bones grow wider. In a slightly more complex way they also grow longer. In one of the body's long bones, such as the femur, or thighbone, development of the sort that makes a 21-inch infant lengthen into a 6-foot adult goes on in knobby ends, where growth discs make new bone matrix. Through complicated chemical processes involving glandular secretions working with the osteoclasts and osteoblasts, the outer face of each growth disc manufactures new cartilage. The inner face replaces the cartilage that is already there with bone; in the process the growth disc pushes itself out to where it will make more bone.

The bones generally stop lengthening in the mid-teens in girls, and somewhat later—about age 20—in boys. But bones never stop the growing process. Perhaps the most surprising thing about them is that they are constantly remaking themselves. Those cells that built the skeleton in the first place continue to work during adulthood and into old age, gradually renewing and replacing bones—at varying rates of speed—so as to keep them as resilient as possible.

To sustain this growth, the body must be supplied enough of certain substances in food: the minerals calcium and phosphorus, and vitamin D.

Calcium from dairy products and leafy vegetables, and phosphorus from eggs, meat and cereal products—digested by the stomach and passed into body fluids through the intestinal walls—reach the bones in the body fluids and are then deposited in the bone by a process called mineralization, which creates crystals of calcium phosphate in the bone matrix, to provide substance and strength. A long-term lack of calcium may contribute to a condition known as osteoporosis, in which the bones become brittle and susceptible to breakage (Chapter 5).

Even with sufficient calcium and phosphorus supplies, the process of mineralization can break down if the body does not get enough vitamin D. There are actually several forms of D vitamins: Some come ready-to-use in foods, but others must be activated by ultraviolet light—this is why vitamin D is called the sunshine vitamin. The curious connection between sunshine and strong bones was not explained until the discovery of the vitamin in 1921, although evidence of a link had been waiting to be recognized for centuries.

Eradicating a childhood crippler

By 1650 physicians in England noticed a disease that came to be called rickets. Children's bones failed to harden in the normal way, remaining soft like cartilage and eventually bending under the weight of growing bodies; the children were left with bowed legs or knock-knees. It became a plague all over Europe as the Industrial Revolution advanced; in the 18th Century 90 per cent of the children in Eastern European cities were victims. Because rickets at first seemed to occur most among children in the smoky, crowded streets of city slums, where sanitation was poor, infection was blamed. But soon it became apparent that wealthy children, who were kept indoors in schools and playrooms, safe from contagion, were even more prone to rickets than the street urchins.

Finally, in the 20th Century two discoveries came almost simultaneously: Rickets was recognized as a deficiency disease caused by a lack of one of the newly found essential vitamins, vitamin D; and vitamin D was seen to be activated when ultraviolet light reached cells in the skin. Rickets was common in the northern cities of Europe because they received less sunlight than southern cities, and even that weak sunlight often was blocked by city smoke and haze.

With the recognition of the cause, rickets was quickly

Bones, muscles and joints working in supreme harmony

Boiled down to basics, the human body would consist of about eight dollars' worth of chemicals. What makes the body much greater than the sum of its parts is its amazing architecture—an arrangement of bones, muscles and joints strong enough to support its weight, rigid enough to protect soft internal organs, flexible enough to provide the agility that has ensured man's survival.

There are more than 200 bones in the body, and their shapes suggest their functions. The rib cage and breastbone, sturdy and strong, protect such precious internal organs as the heart and lungs. The bones of the hands and fingers, tapered and small, seem meant for fine manipulations. Joints, like the bones that come together to form them, are constructed to suit the tasks they perform *(page 19)*. The neck is equipped with a pivot that allows the head to twist side to side, the shoulder with a ball-and-socket joint for motion in a full circle.

The body's more than 600 muscles also come in various shapes and sizes, yet they work in a single way—by contracting *(overleaf)*. Together, bones, muscles and joints work in harmony to make the human animal supreme on earth.

How the human skeleton gives unparalleled versatility is suggsted by the running figure at right. Bones in legs and feet help support, balance and propel; curves in the spine help absorb shocks; hard bones of the rib cage and skull protect vital organs. All combine to support man's unique upright stance.

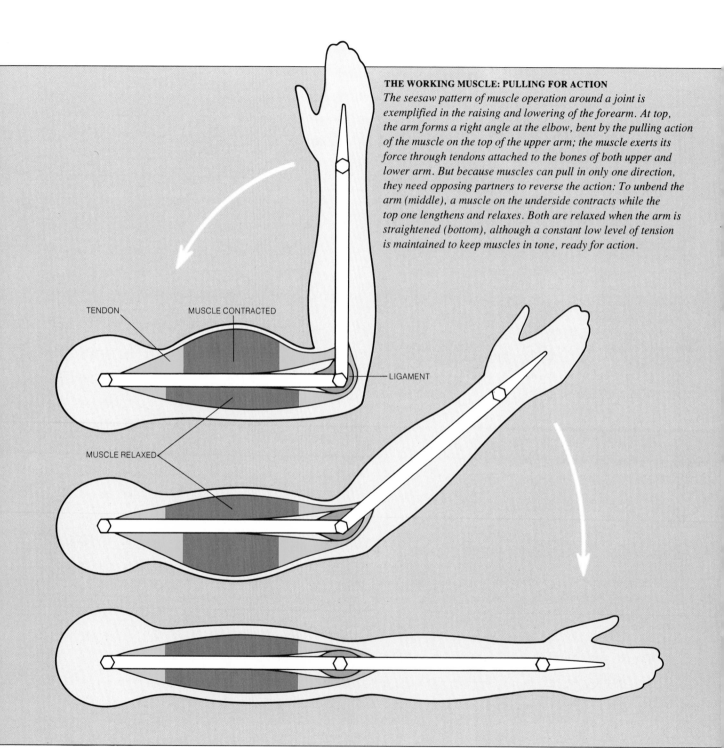

THE WORKING MUSCLE: PULLING FOR ACTION
The seesaw pattern of muscle operation around a joint is exemplified in the raising and lowering of the forearm. At top, the arm forms a right angle at the elbow, bent by the pulling action of the muscle on the top of the upper arm; the muscle exerts its force through tendons attached to the bones of both upper and lower arm. But because muscles can pull in only one direction, they need opposing partners to reverse the action: To unbend the arm (middle), a muscle on the underside contracts while the top one lengthens and relaxes. Both are relaxed when the arm is straightened (bottom), although a constant low level of tension is maintained to keep muscles in tone, ready for action.

TENDON

MUSCLE CONTRACTED

LIGAMENT

MUSCLE RELAXED

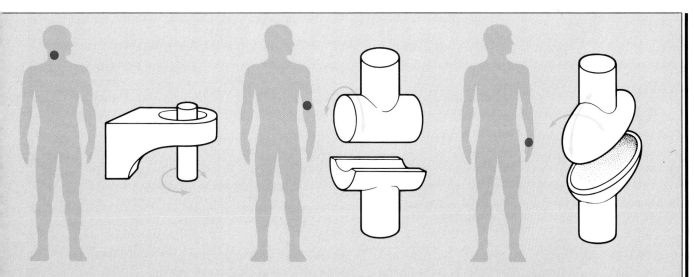

A JOINT THAT PIVOTS SIDE TO SIDE
Rotation of one bone within another is allowed by a pivot joint, such as one atop the spine. There, a bony ring from one spinal segment encircles a peglike projection from a second, permitting the head to turn.

THE HINGE JOINT: ONE-WAY MOVEMENT
Strong and mobile, a hinge joint operates in much the same fashion as the hinge on a door, swinging back and forth, but not from side to side. The elbow is a hinge joint, and so is the knee.

THE ELLIPSOID JOINT: AN EGG IN A SPOON
Like an egg resting in a spoon, the oval ellipsoid joint provides limited motion in two directions. In the wrist it permits the hand to move up and down and side to side, but not to rotate completely.

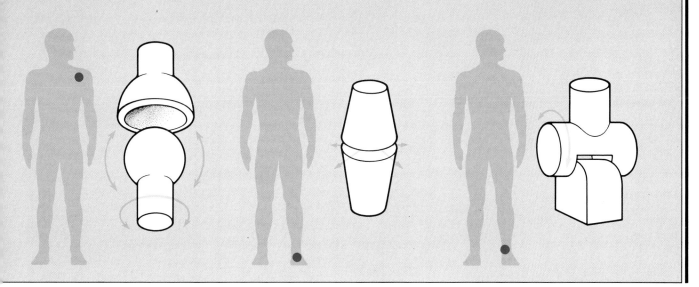

THE VERSATILE BALL-AND-SOCKET JOINT
Most flexible are the ball-and-socket joints: The spherical end of one bone fits a cuplike socket on the other to allow circular motion, even completely around. It gives maximum mobility to shoulder and hip.

THE GLIDING JOINT: LIMITED TRAVEL
The simplest movement between bones occurs in a gliding joint, where one bone slides partway across another. Surrounding structures restrict the motion. Gliding joints connect small bones in hands and feet.

THE SADDLE JOINT: TWO-PLANE MOVEMENT
The saddle joint, as in the ankle, is shaped to permit combinations of limited movements along perpendicular planes. Hence the ankle allows the foot to turn inward slightly as it swivels up and down.

eradicated; by the middle of the 20th Century the disease had essentially disappeared from the industrialized countries. Outdoor activity in sunshine is routine for nearly all children. In addition, babies are given vitamin concentrates, and in the United States milk is required by law to be fortified with vitamin D. In Europe, where such a law does not always exist, doctors give children injections of vitamin D every six weeks to three months to keep them free of rickets, their limbs straight, their bones properly hardened.

It is vital, though, that some cartilage remain in bones, particularly at the ends. There it not only plays a role in bone growth, but it provides a soft, pliable cushion for the meeting of two bones at the connectors called joints.

How bones are connected

Some joints simply act as meeting points for bones that do not move; the joints of the skull compress slightly during birth and then, their job done, solidify and lock together, their serrated edges fitting neatly into each other to protect the brain. Some joints consist of little more than cartilage and move hardly at all: Those between ribs and breastbone, for example, allow just enough movement for breathing. Similarly, in the female pelvis there are four normally rigid joints that manage to become slightly flexible during childbirth, helping to ease the passage of the baby. Most joints, however, move with remarkable dexterity in their unending assignment of keeping the body flexible.

Designed to permit movement between bones that must meet but not touch each other, the joints are masterpieces of engineering. They must bind the two or more bones to each other firmly, cushion them against each other and lubricate them adequately so that they will continue to meet the demands of the muscles for a lifetime—lifting packages, swinging golf clubs, walking. It was extraordinary conditioning of the joints that enabled circus aerialist Lillian Leitzel to rotate her shoulder and arm so that she could whip herself over a rope like an airplane propeller for 249 turns.

The simplest type of joint is the hinge joint, which works exactly like a door hinge, moving neither sideways nor backward: Fingers can double themselves to make a fist but cannot be bent backward (except by some extremely flexible persons). Akin to the hinge but slightly more complicated is the rotary, or pivot, joint, exemplified by the elbows: Although it is basically a hinge, the elbow joint also permits the two bones of the forearm to cross over each other on command so that you may go from palms-up to palms-down.

The most versatile is the ball-and-socket joint, in which the round end of one bone fits into the cup-shaped end of another. The shoulder ball-and-socket arrangement is the most maneuverable in the body, a fact that would not be denied by traffic officers, ball players and symphony conductors, all of whom benefit from the circular moves it permits. There are many variations.

The saddle joint allows movement in two planes: The thumb, for example, can move toward the fingers to grasp something and can also align with the index finger to flatten the hand for a military salute. The gliding joint merely lets one bone move across another in almost any direction. The wrist contains 34 such joints, linking its eight marvelously dovetailed bones. ''The narrowest hinge on my hand,'' Walt Whitman remarked, ''puts to scorn all machinery.''

Although their construction varies, most joints are made up of the same elements. The joint is enclosed in a tough, fibrous capsule of connective tissue, which secretes a liquid—synovial fluid—that lubricates the moving parts. Thus the entire affair is much like a sealed bearing in a car. Outside this capsule the fibrous anchors called ligaments surround the joint and link the two bones, protecting the capsule and helping to keep any motion of the joint within safe limits. And where the muscle tissues called tendons or sinews pass alongside a large joint, linking a muscle on one side to a bone on the other, small fluid-filled pouches, or bursae, also act as buffers. For example, in the knee—a joint subject to much stress—there are 13 cushioning bursae.

The larger tendons often stand out clearly over the joint they span, as do those behind the knee. Smaller tendons can be seen at work on the back of a clenching fist: The fingers have no muscle in them but are governed instead by the muscles of the palm and forearm that pull on the tendons. Herman Melville, the American novelist, observed, ''The human body indeed is like a ship; its bones being the stiff standing-rigging, and the sinews the small running ropes, that manage all the motions.''

Maintaining muscle power

The bones and sinews manage the motions of the body, but muscles create the motions. At the same time they are nodding the head, flexing an arm or stretching the mouth into a smile, muscles are circulating blood, expelling breath, digesting food and operating every other vital organ in the body. By converting chemical energy from food to mechanical energy, they sustain the pulse of existence. Of the 600 or so muscles that gird the human skeleton and keep it running, there are three kinds: heart muscle, which pumps the blood an average of 70 times a minute, 40 million times a year, for a lifetime; smooth muscle, which unceasingly conducts blood, urine and other fluids throughout the body's systems, nudges nutrients through the stomach and intestines, widens or narrows the eye's pupil and makes skin hair stand on end by creating gooseflesh; and skeletal muscle, the kind that can be seen rippling under the skin, most notably in the biceps.

Although skeletal muscles are sometimes called voluntary muscles because they react on command, while smooth ones are named involuntary because they generally operate without conscious control, the designations are misleading, because the dividing line between them is inexact. Your eyelids can be blinked at will, yet most of the time they blink by themselves. The tongue is a voluntary muscle, yet when you swallow, it automatically rises to the roof of the mouth to close off your throat and form a chute; and when the jaws snap shut the tongue almost always (the exceptions can hurt) gets out of the way. Many of the ordinarily involuntary muscles can be controlled consciously—people can even learn to slow their heart rate or lower their blood pressure.

Muscles do their work by contracting—pulling. They never push. Because they only pull—as sailors do on rigging—it takes a pair of them to permit a range of movement. To raise a coffee cup, the biceps muscle in the front contracts and the triceps in the back of the arm keeps the cup from smashing into the mouth; to lower the cup, the triceps tugs gently while the biceps lets go equally gently, preventing the cup from plummeting to the table.

So precise is this control that many muscles can be coordinated to perform an action at varying speeds. A tennis player can start a serve slowly, then once at the top of the serve, smash the ball suddenly, completing the arm's circle of movement—a symphony of complex, modulated muscular exertion involving almost every section of the body.

This tennis player can control muscles so completely because of the way they are constructed and sparked into action. Each muscle consists of great numbers of tiny string-like fibers—each in turn composed of bundles of infinitesimal filaments—that vary in length from half an inch to about a foot. Small muscles have just a few fibers, large ones a great many; altogether there are some six trillion muscle fibers in the body, each no thicker than a hair but each capable of supporting 1,000 times its weight. When the tennis player decides to lob a ball over the net, his brain sends out nerve impulses that activate the fibers of the appropriate muscle, one motor nerve generally controlling a number of fibers. When a fiber is activated, it responds instantly and completely, pulling at full strength. Yet the action remains controlled because the brain selects the number of fibers to go into action and determines their frequency of operation: Each fiber pulls at full force but for only a fraction of a second.

The more any muscle is used, the stronger it becomes. The effort makes the heart supply more blood and nutrients, stimulating the growth of new muscle fibers and blood vessels. Thus exercise will enlarge and strengthen muscles as it does bones. And specific exercises can be used to improve certain muscles—those in the stomach to aid lifting, those in the legs and shoulders to avoid sprains or strains.

The human frame requires only simple care to maintain its marvelous agility and power. Regular activity keeps bones and muscles in constant, strengthening growth. A sensible diet—one that balances minerals, vitamins and the other components of everyday foods—sustains growth and energizes muscles. And knowing how this framework operates—while understanding the limits beyond which it cannot be pushed—will help you safeguard it for a lifetime. ❋

Making crippled children whole

A revolution in the treatment of crippled children has now made defects in bone structure less a life-darkening tragedy than a temporary obstacle. No longer must such youngsters face permanent disability and isolation. Twisted spines can be straightened, dislocated hips reset, misshapen feet rebuilt. Even children lacking legs can be made to walk.

At the heart of the revolution is early detection, for a defect found early, before it causes distortion of other parts of the anatomy, is easier to treat. In almost all hospitals today, doctors gently examine newborns' hips and feet for signs of loose hip joints or clubfoot, a deformity in which the foot is twisted inward.

Along with early detection have come radical advances in treatment. Hips that slip out of joint can often be cured with an unobtrusive harness *(page 28),* instead of the immobilizing body cast once required. For the sideways spinal curve of scoliosis, there are new lightweight braces, too, as well as improved surgical techniques. In one method, a metal rod is implanted and fastened to the backbone to straighten it. For the one child in a thousand born with clubfoot, delicate manipulations pull toe and foot bones and muscles into line; a surgeon sometimes provides the finishing touch, making cuts in ligaments and tendons to allow them to lengthen so bones can grow normally.

For children without legs, artificial limbs of lightweight metal and plastic have begun to replace heavier, wood-and-metal models. New artificial arms and hands imitate natural appearance and function: The soft plastic hand of one model requires less precise positioning and less strength to operate, making grasping easier. With devices and techniques such as these, the child born with a structural defect can expect to grow up to a normal life.

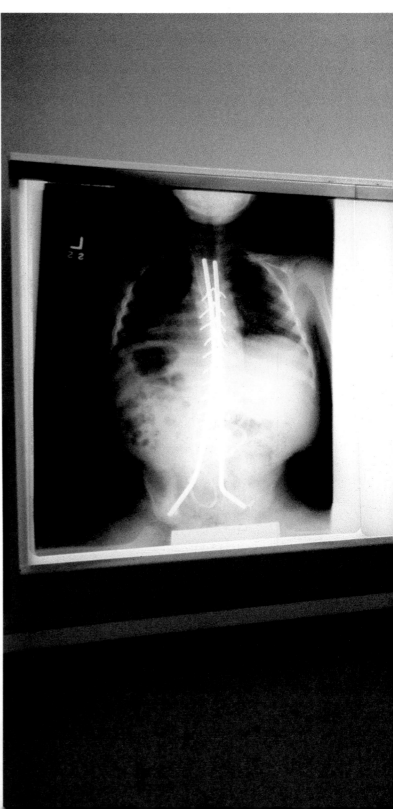

Seated on Dr. Ron Ellis' knee, five-year-old John McGuigan looks over X-rays taken after surgery that corrected his scoliosis (curved spine). In the operation, at Children's Hospital of Philadelphia, a metal rod was attached permanently to his backbone, wires hugging each vertebra. The device is seen as white lines in both the rear view (left) and the side view (right).

PHOTOGRAPHS BY LINDA BARTLETT

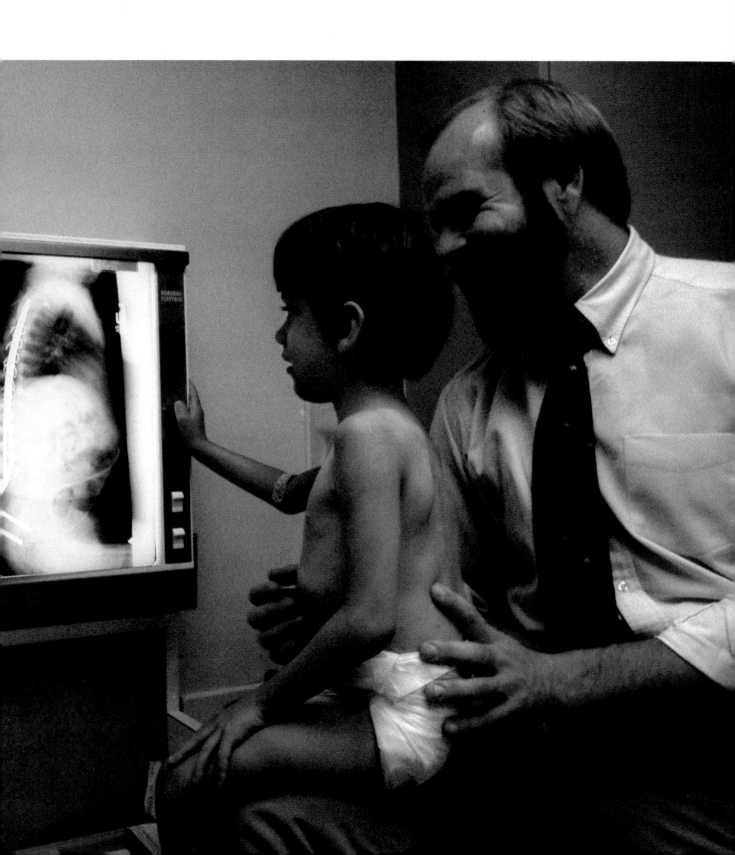

Straightening a twisted spine

The twisted spine called scoliosis can not only deform a
child's body but so cramp the rib cage that it interferes with
breathing. Today the curvature can usually be halted by a
brace *(below)*. Experiments with electricity show promise,
stimulating muscles on the convex side of the curve so that
they contract and hold the spine in line *(right)*. And now the
twist can be partially straightened by cutting the back open,
implanting a steel rod and fastening it to vertebrae so that it
forces the spine more nearly upright and holds it that way;
meanwhile bone grafts fuse the vertebrae, welding the spine
permanently into this form.

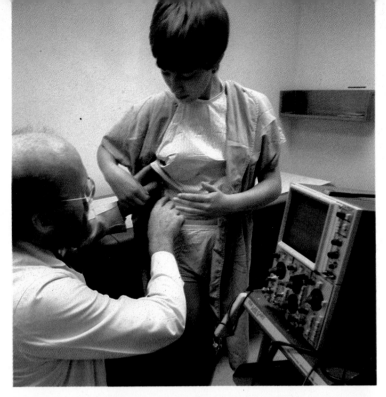

*Dr. Hugh Watts tapes electrodes of an electrical stimulator
to the skin of Hannah Barrett, a teenager with moderate
scoliosis. The device strengthens muscles to stop curvature.*

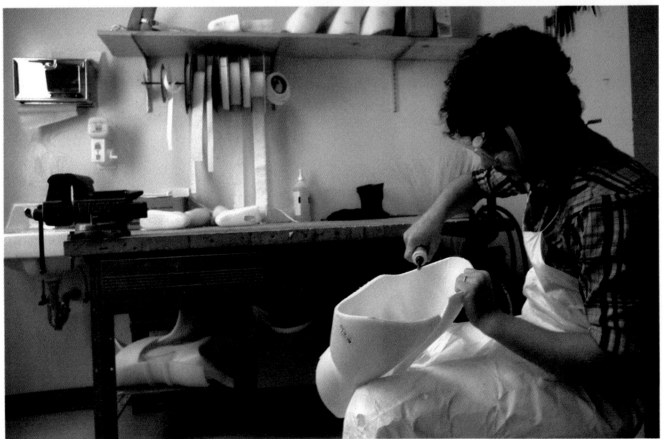

*Wearing goggles to protect his eyes from
flying bits of plastic, a technician in the
hospital shop smooths the edges of a
lightweight brace. Braces like this one,
weighing no more than three pounds,
replace heavier metal-and-leather types.*

*Bill Penney, head of the brace shop, checks the fit of a back
brace worn by 13-year-old Debbie Benson. She is required to
wear the pelvis-to-underarm brace 23 hours a day—removing
it only to bathe—until her bones reach maturity.*

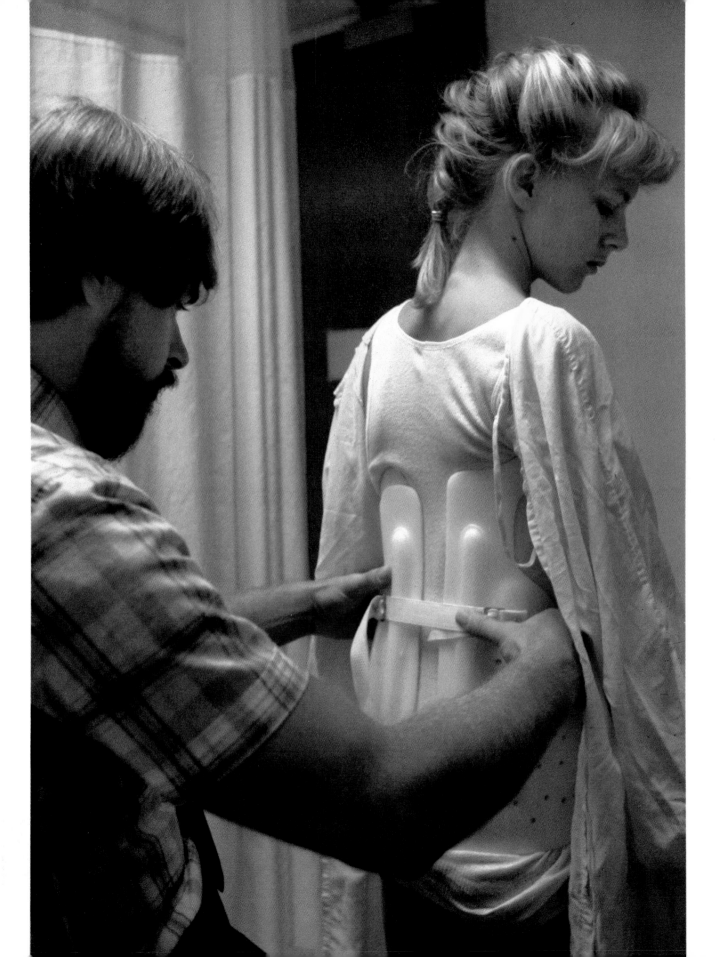

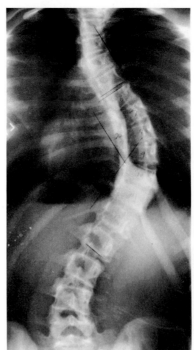
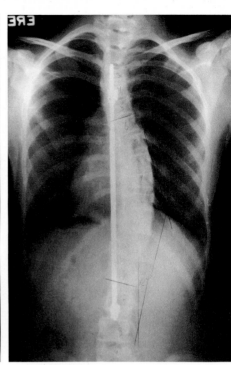

"Before" and "after" X-rays of a scoliosis-afflicted spine reveal the twofold reduction in curvature achieved by a rigid rod wired to the spine at top and bottom—the straight white line in the center of the right-hand X-ray.

Diane Hazel, who has had a rod inserted along her spine to control curvature, lies draped on a frame while Dr. Malcolm L. Ecker molds a fiberglass cast. Her face is covered for protection from debris; the cast will help keep her spine straight.

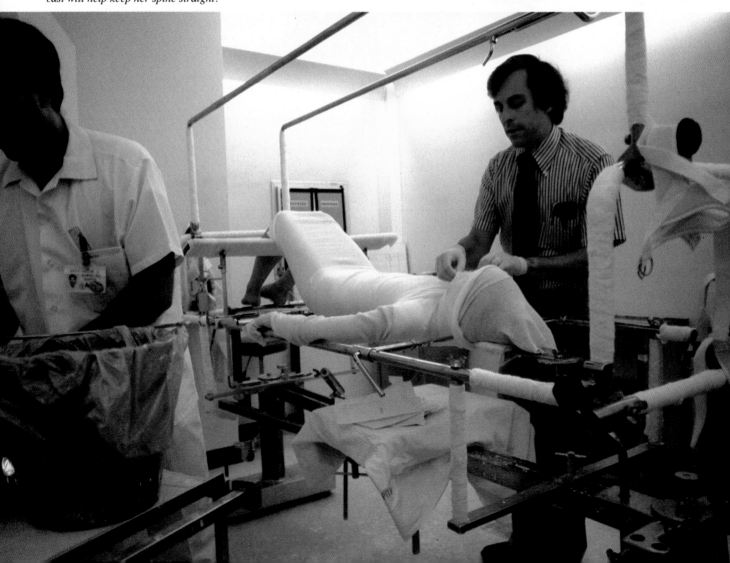

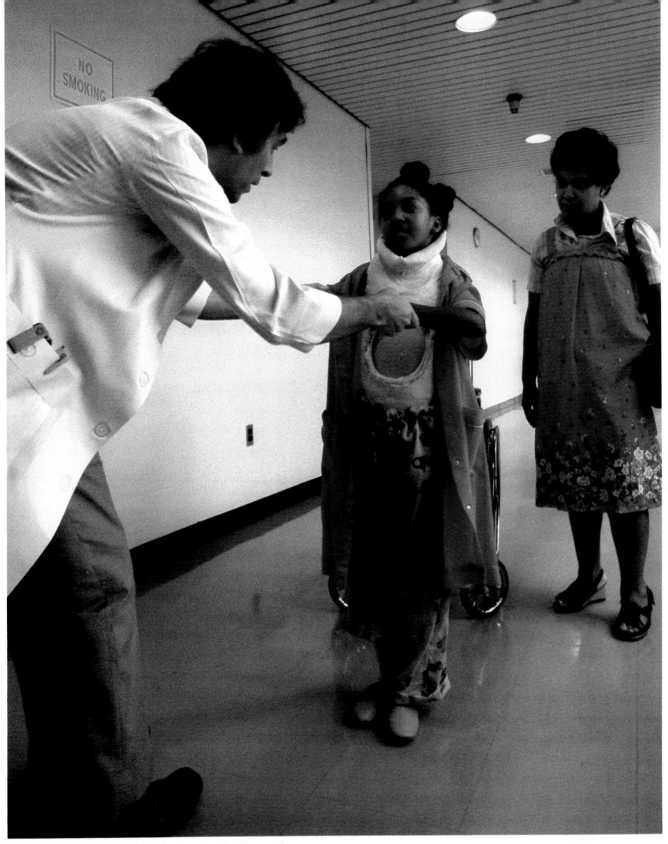

*Just a week after spine-straightening surgery, Joy Derry takes
her first steps, encouraged by Dr. Ecker and her mother. The 10-
year-old also suffers from heart disease; the hole in her cast
allows her chest to expand freely, helping her breathe more easily
and making it possible to avoid extra strain on her heart.*

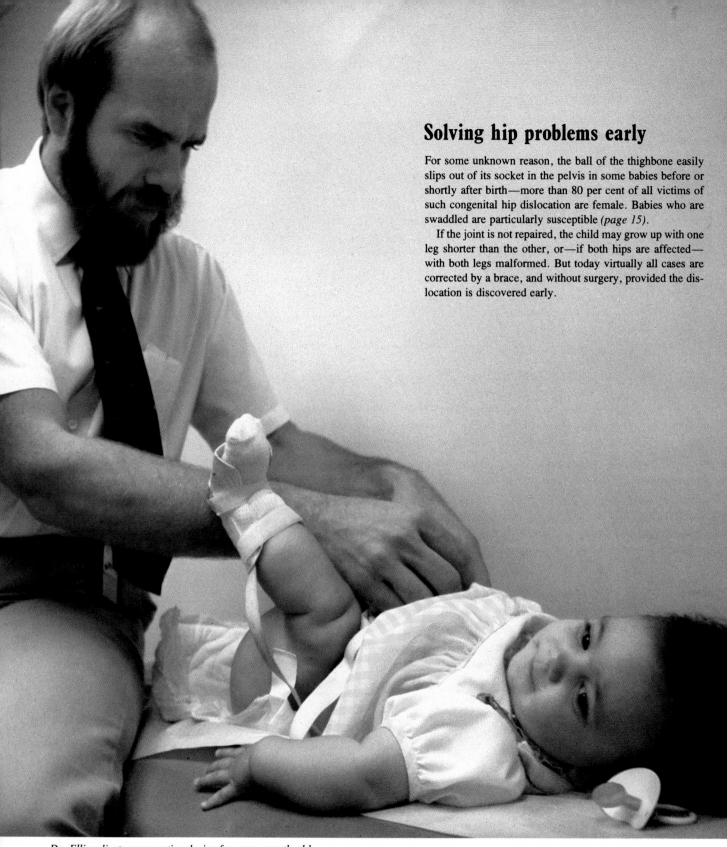

Solving hip problems early

For some unknown reason, the ball of the thighbone easily slips out of its socket in the pelvis in some babies before or shortly after birth—more than 80 per cent of all victims of such congenital hip dislocation are female. Babies who are swaddled are particularly susceptible *(page 15)*.

If the joint is not repaired, the child may grow up with one leg shorter than the other, or—if both hips are affected—with both legs malformed. But today virtually all cases are corrected by a brace, and without surgery, provided the dislocation is discovered early.

Dr. Ellis adjusts a corrective device for seven-month-old Monique La Perriere, who was born with a dislocated hip. Until she is about a year old, Monique must wear the canvas harness, held in place by shoulder straps and a chest band, to keep her hips flexed upward and her legs apart. Formerly, an infant with that problem would have been put in a confining body cast.

To make sure a possible hip dislocation is detected early enough for treatment, Dr. Russ Windsor bends a newborn girl's knees and feels the position of her hip joints. Such screening is now routine in virtually all American hospitals.

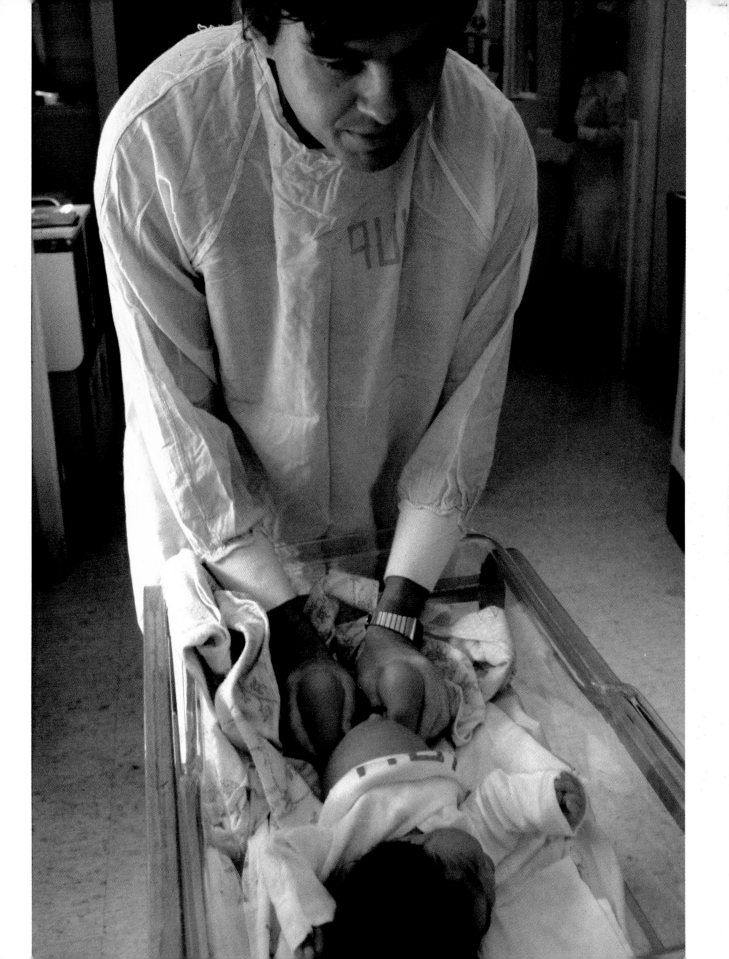

How to change the shape of a foot

Abnormal walking patterns such as severe toeing in or out usually are not seen until a child begins to toddle at about a year old. But even then, bones are still only partly formed from soft cartilage, and nonsurgical therapy *(below)* suffices.

A worse problem is clubfoot, blamed by some authorities on malformed muscles that pull the foot awry. To mold a twisted foot into a normal form, orthopedists stretch and press foot bones and muscles into shape, then set the foot in a cast, repeating the procedure weekly for as long as a year. Most children learn to walk and run without impairment.

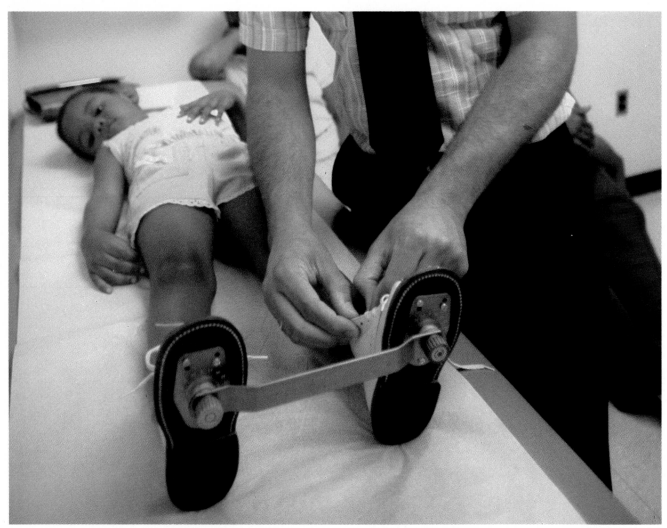

A resident at Children's Hospital of Philadelphia adjusts three-year-old Nadira Lynch's sleeping bar, a device the child wears in bed to correct her gait—she walks with knees turned in and toes pointed out. The bar holds Nadira's knees apart and keeps her toes pointed straight ahead.

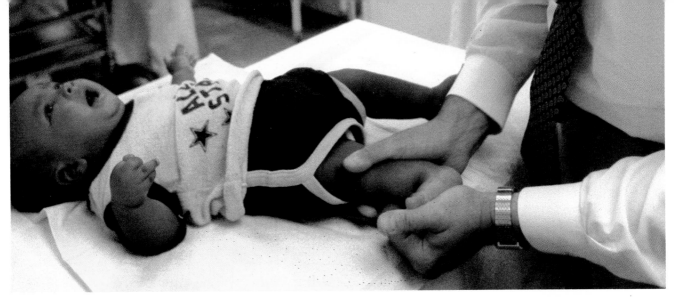

Five-month-old Antoine Garnett, born with a clubfoot, breathes hard as Dr. Ronald Pitkow gently moves bones and muscles to align the foot.

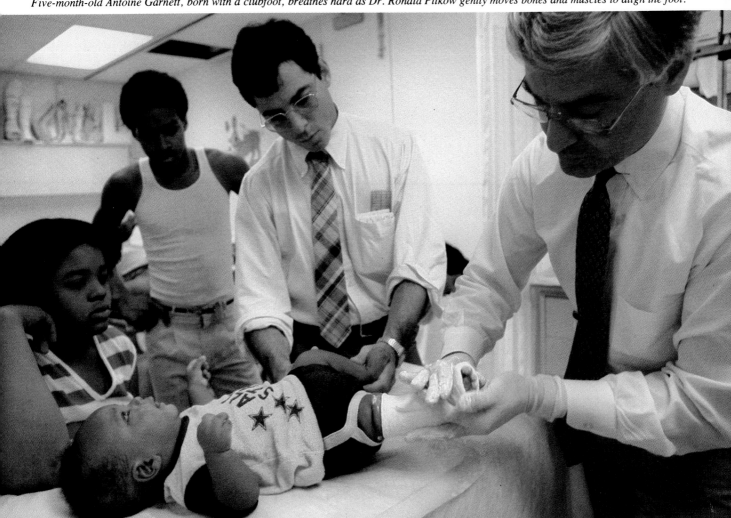

Antoine's parents watch while a resident helps Dr. Pitkow mold a plaster cast. The cast maintains the shape the doctor has attained by manipulation. Antoine returns to the hospital's Foot and Gait Clinic every week to have his foot reshaped and recast; eventually surgery will make final adjustments.

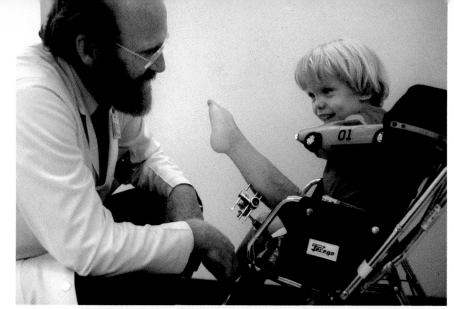

Grinning Matty Purington, aged three, holds a toy car with his congenitally shortened arm as Dr. Watts examines a temporary system to straighten his leg, also malformed. The temporary support will later be replaced by leg braces to help Matty meet his goal: "I'm going to walk!"

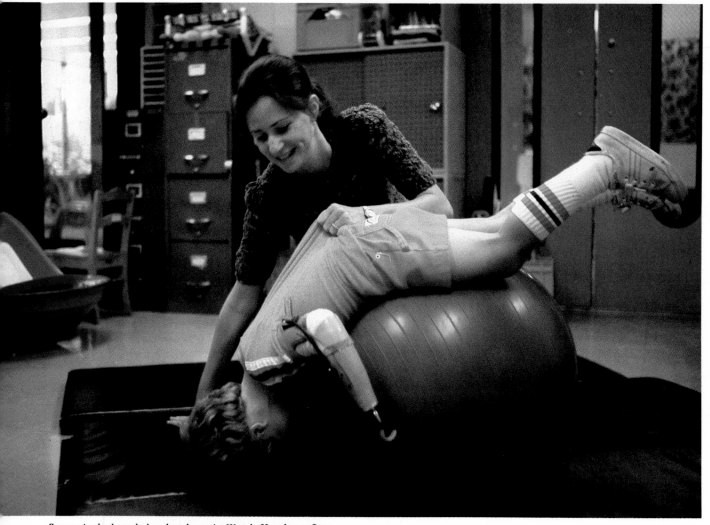

Secure in the knowledge that therapist Wendy Hart has a firm grip on his shirt, five-year-old Jesse Nariskus rolls over a large rubber ball. To do this, Jesse must use both arms for balance, including the artificial arm and hook hand he has worn since he was six months old. Play therapy such as this helps Jesse build confidence and encourages him to use his prosthesis actively.

New limbs for new lives

In the past, many youngsters missing part of an arm or leg—from birth defect or through accident—were allowed to flounder without mechanical aid until they reached school age. And then they might be given a cut-down adult artificial limb, ill-fitting and clumsy.

Today artificial limbs, or prostheses, are not only made to fit all ages, but they incorporate improvements once only dreamed of. Legs, for example, have hydraulic knee joints, which imitate natural movement and give control over walking speed—impossible with a simple hinge joint.

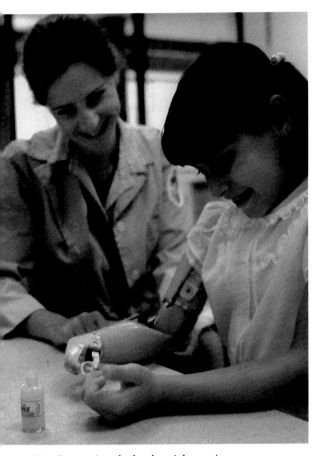

Tina Brocaccio, who lost her right arm in an automobile accident, puts on nail polish with an artificial replacement, attached at her chest and neck. The hand opens and closes in response to shoulder muscles.

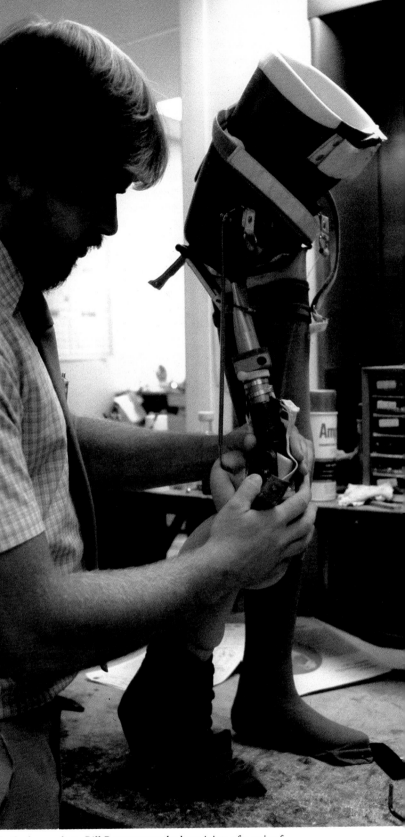

In the brace shop, Bill Penney tests the knee joints of a pair of child-sized artificial legs. The knees bend when the wearer moves his trunk muscles; the apparatus by the right thigh is operated by hand and locks and unlocks the legs for standing and sitting. The foam padding and the dark stockings tailor the prosthesis to its owner, Frankie Rankins (overleaf).

34

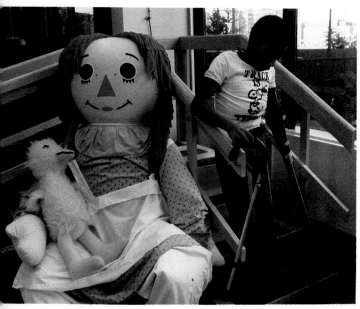

Too busy to be distracted by a larger-than-life rag doll, Frankie Rankins, born missing an arm and both legs, practices walking down stairs on his man-made legs with the aid of a cane and a crutch that screws into his prosthetic arm. Eventually Frankie will become proficient enough with his legs to be able to give up the crutch and walk using only the cane.

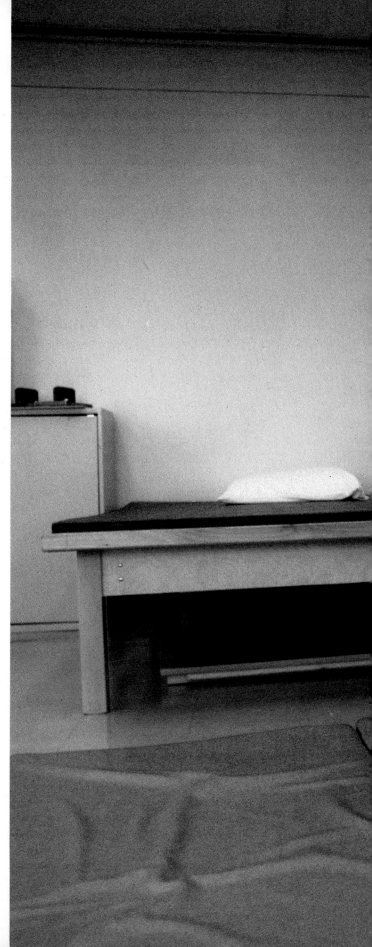

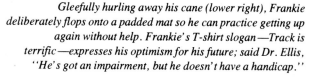

Gleefully hurling away his cane (lower right), Frankie deliberately flops onto a padded mat so he can practice getting up again without help. Frankie's T-shirt slogan—Track is terrific—expresses his optimism for his future; said Dr. Ellis, "He's got an impairment, but he doesn't have a handicap."

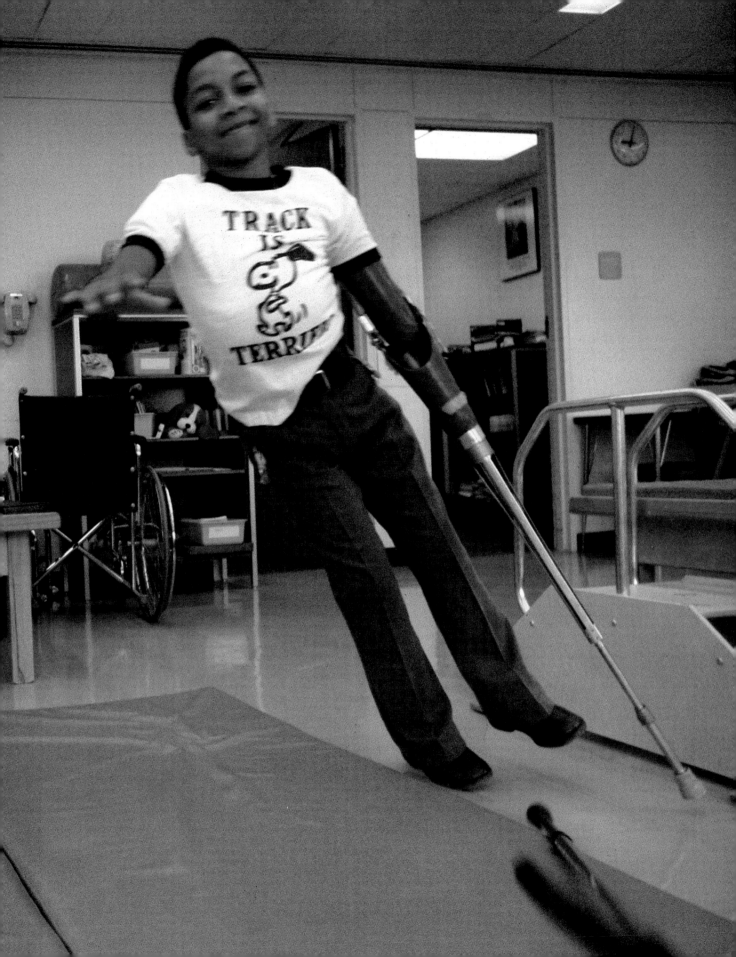

Beating a bad back

"Oh, my aching back!" The cry is all but universal. Eight out of 10 people on earth can expect that, at some time, they will suffer the effects of backache, ranging from painful annoyance to total disability. Many will meet it in the most bewildering circumstances, and without apparent warning.

As writer J. D. Reed was walking through New York City's Pennsylvania Station on the way to his commuter train, he sneezed. Suddenly he found himself on all fours. Unable to stand, he crawled aboard the train, rode homeward on his hands and knees and had to be carried to his doctor's office for relief of the spasm that had doubled him up. The chairman of a major corporation leaned down to pick up a dropped pencil during a board meeting and felt a violent contraction in his back. Unable to move, he was carried to the doctor in his hunched-over position. San Francisco house-wife Barbara Gordon, stricken while working in her attic, lay there for eight agonizing hours before being discovered.

Such bizarre attacks are neither rare nor unpredictable. Reed himself later wrote: "I was disappointed to learn that my case was so ordinary." He had suffered a massive and abrupt contraction of the muscles, a spasm so powerful that the muscles locked, unable to relax again. A spasm is the typical response of an overworked back to tension and fatigue. A week before that sneeze immobilized him, Reed had put his overweight and out-of-shape body through a strenuous game of squash. At the end of the match, he had felt twinges in his lower spine—sure signals, he later learned, that he was a "No. 1 candidate for back pain."

Candidates like Reed are part of a crowded field. In the United States alone, some 70 million people suffer from back pain severe enough to require medical treatment; another two million join the ranks each year. Their agonies exact a staggering financial and social toll. In a recent year more than 90 million workdays were lost to back disorders, some five billion dollars were spent on treatment for back pain, and workers were paid an estimated nine billion dollars in compensation for on-the-job back injuries—more than the cost for all other work-related ailments combined.

Anyone stricken by backache is in fashionable as well as abundant company: Presidents and potentates, movie stars and literary lights, even superbly conditioned athletes are fellow victims. Author Ernest Hemingway, like many sufferers, found it painful simply to sit down; he wrote standing up. President John F. Kennedy used a rocking chair to ease his pain. And tennis champion Tracy Austin was sidelined for four and a half months in 1981 by low-back pain and a pinched nerve that caused piercing pains in the buttocks.

Back pain is hardly new—people have been complaining about their backs since man began the extraordinary balancing act of standing erect. Anthropologists have found spinal disorders in the 100,000-year-old human skeletons of the Neanderthals who preceded modern man. The ancient Egyptians and Greeks left records of remedies for back pain.

Then as now, ideas for treatment were often in conflict. Hippocrates, the greatest physician of ancient Greece, took what would now be considered a conservative approach. He

Light beamed through a grid produces Moiré patterns, tracing back contours that might reveal spinal curvature. Depending on how far the light waves travel, some interfere with one another to create dark wavy lines. The contours pictured are normal.

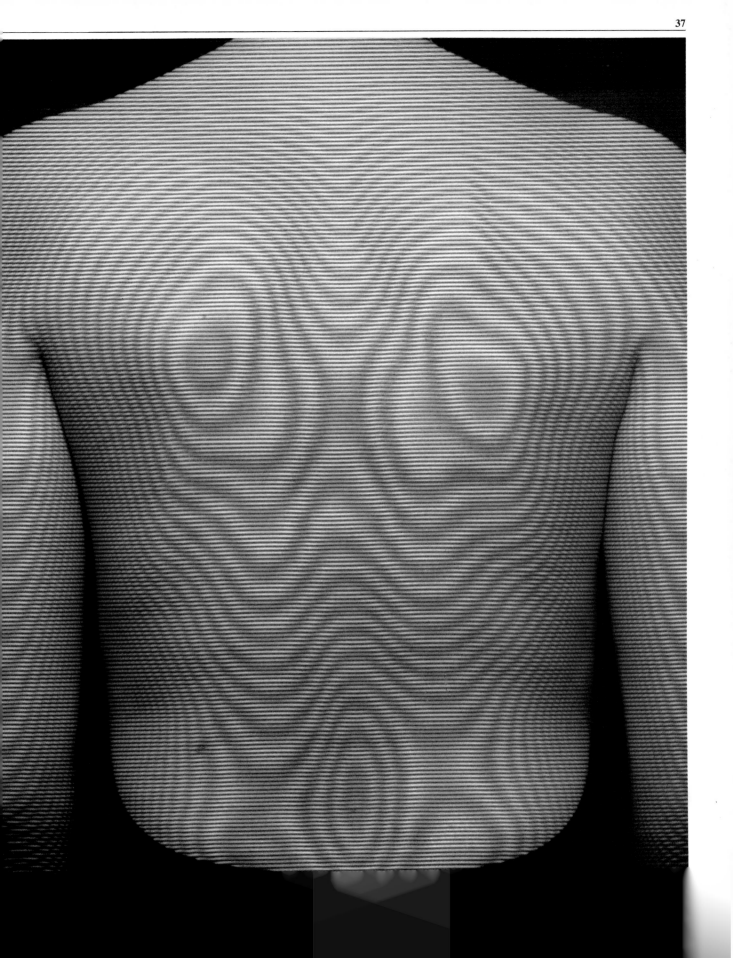

argued that physicians could do little to treat ordinary back-aches beyond counseling patients to rest so that the healing forces of nature could do their work. For severe cases, he suggested a rude form of traction, in which the patient was immobilized face down on a board while secured with straps around the ankles, knees, pelvis and armpits.

Then as now, there was no dearth of unorthodox treatments. In one, the sufferer was fastened to a ladder, upended and either dropped to the ground or shaken vigorously up and down to loosen the vertebrae. Hippocrates, like his modern counterparts, cautioned against such dangerous quackery, observing that the ladder technique was "principally practiced by those physicians who seek to astonish the mob."

Today there is even less agreement on cures for backache. Osteopaths, chiropractors, biofeedback technicians, acupuncturists, peddlers of exotic drugs—all offer their own theories and therapies. Comedian Joe E. Lewis used to tell of the time he fell prey to a particularly severe attack. He went to see his doctor, who advised him to apply hot towels. On the way home, Lewis stopped for dinner at his favorite restaurant, and the headwaiter there assured him that cold towels worked better. Later Lewis confronted his doctor with the news. "That's funny," said the perplexed physician. "The headwaiter at the country club told me to use hot towels."

Orthopedic surgeons, who are the accepted medical authorities on back pain, go along with both waiters. They recommend heat *and* cold—at different times, depending on the injury and its state of healing *(page 94)*. They also continue to seek alternatives to the old folk remedies and the new surgical and chemical weapons that make up the arsenal of conventional medicine. Most of them agree that no known drug can cure common backache—although some may ease its symptoms—and an ever-growing group believe that the spinal surgery done on some 200,000 Americans each year is in many cases unnecessary and in some harmful.

But the picture is not hopeless. The most effective cure for backache, and the best protection against it, are already built into your body. Generally, both prevention and cure lie in the muscles that hold your spine erect. If you keep these muscles in good condition and use them prudently, your back will

function without pain. And if your back does develop trouble, you can usually diagnose the cause, ease the pain and prevent a recurrence. Only when certain readily identifiable signs point to a severe problem need you call a doctor.

How to avoid an aching back

One important step in preventing back pain is learning to recognize and avoid the back-threatening situations of 20th Century life. Among the most insidious is simply sitting in a chair. "Modern furniture is the worst thing that ever happened to most backs," wrote Dr. Marilyn Moffat of New York University. Big, low, soft chairs force the back to heroic efforts just to get into and out of them. Even sitting still in such a chair is perilous: Pressure on your lower back can be about twice as great as it is when you are standing.

The best chair is fairly straight, supports the small of your back, and puts your knees slightly higher than your hips. A chair with arms is even better, for resting your arms upon them relaxes the muscles of your upper back. Steer clear of high stools, which allow your legs to dangle and force you to arch your back for balance. (For pictorial directions on the right way to sit in a chair or an automobile, see page 62).

Unlike modern chairs, modern bedding generally poses no threat to the back. Contrary to popular myth, you need not sleep on a rock-hard bed to protect your back; an inner-spring mattress on a box spring provides adequate support for your body. The only true problem bed is one with a sag so pronounced that it bends your spine into an unnatural curve. Shore up a sagging mattress by placing beneath it a bedboard, either a piece of plywood or the kind of inexpensive folding bedboard, available at pharmacies and surgical supply houses, that many chronic back sufferers use.

In addition to avoiding hazardous furniture, train yourself to stand, move and lift loads in ways that relieve your spine of the stress caused by overarching the back *(pages 60-62)*. Wear flat shoes whenever possible; high heels tilt the pelvis backward, causing a stressful swayback.

Ultimately, the best defense against backache is a set of strong back muscles. Ten minutes a day spent on exercises not only strengthens the back against everyday strains, but builds up a reserve of strength, a kind of muscular bank account on which to draw when you subject your back to such special strains as lifting a child out of a crib or a heavy package from the trunk of a car. Equally good are sports that call for endurance and provide all-over conditioning—walking, bicycling and some styles of jogging and swimming.

However, some sports—including some of the most popular—subject the spine to potentially harmful stresses. Canadian orthopedist Hamilton Hall classified these activities into three types: weight-loading, rotation-causing and back-arching. Weight-loading sports, which tend to compress the spine, include not only weight lifting itself, but bowling, horseback riding, motorbiking and jogging on a hard surface. Rotation-causing activities subject the spine to a forceful twist; among them are squash, racquetball, tennis, batting in baseball or softball, and golf. Novice skiers may also twist their spines (experienced skiers learn to swivel their legs and are less likely to wrench their backs), but skiing generally belongs in the back-arching class, along with tennis, badminton, volleyball, basketball, rowing, archery and two swimming strokes, the breast stroke and the butterfly.

The best way to guard against the ill effects of these sports is to limber and stretch your back with exercises before you go jogging or head for the playing field. This precaution is vital for weekend enthusiasts; every Monday morning, orthopedists' offices are filled with weekend warriors whose backs were not up to the strain of their favorite sport.

Back-strengthening exercises can be crucial during pregnancy. To protect a pregnant woman's spine against the weight of a developing baby, obstetricians often suggest rehabilitation-type back exercises and teach the patient the correct ways of sitting, standing, walking and lifting. They generally advise against high heels, even if such shoes have never caused the woman pain before; during pregnancy, the heels may prove to be a backbreaking last straw.

Finally, back exercises are especially valuable for anyone peculiarly prone to backache. These potential sufferers fall into three classes: those who are disposed to the affliction by heredity, those with congenital irregularities of muscles or bones, and those whose back muscles are woefully out of

shape. A few rule-of-thumb indications can tell you whether you belong in one of these groups.

If several members of your family have a history of chronic back pain, you may have inherited a predisposition to the malady. The most common hereditary time bomb for the back is a weakness in the spine's cushioning discs, which makes these anatomical shock absorbers especially susceptible to everyday wear and tear.

Minor variations in body structure can also cause trouble. Most people have one leg somewhat shorter than the other, for example. A difference great enough to unbalance the body sets up backaches. To see if this applies to you, note whether the heel of one shoe wears down faster; the less-worn heel is on the shorter leg. A simple heel lift, a felt or leather wedge fitted by a shoemaker or bought at a drugstore,

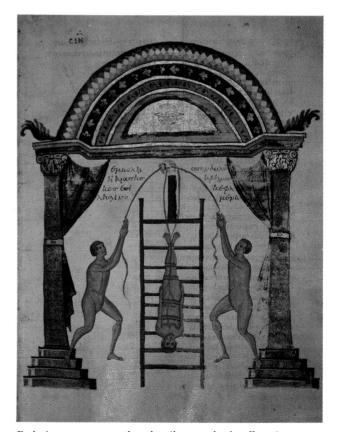

Enduring a cure worse than the ailment, a back sufferer is bound upside down to a ladder, which is then hoisted and dropped, supposedly jolting displaced bones into alignment. The treatment, here depicted in a 10th Century illustration, was first described about 1,500 years earlier by Hippocrates who, like later doctors of repute, regarded the practice with skepticism.

in the shoe of the shorter leg will often correct the imbalance.

To determine whether you have a mild degree of the sideways spinal curvature called scoliosis, stand facing a mirror and look at your lower trunk in the glass—one hipbone higher or more prominent than the other indicates that condition. And to test yourself for excessive arching of the lower spine, stand with your back to a wall or doorframe, with your heels, buttocks, shoulders and head all touching the surface. You should barely be able to slide your hand between the wall and the small of the back; if the space is so large that your hand passes through easily, your back is excessively swayed and you may be vulnerable to backache.

One obvious warning of impending pain comes from the back muscles themselves. If they need strengthening they will signal that fact with frequent twinges. A systematic method of evaluating back strength, used by many doctors, consists of a six-step test developed in pioneering studies of backache victims during the 1940s by Dr. Hans Kraus and his associate Dr. Sonja Weber of the Posture Clinic of Columbia-Presbyterian Hospital in New York City. The Kraus-Weber test is simple to take and score. If any one of its six movements is impossible for you, or if you feel discomfort or pain while performing them, your stomach, hip, thigh or back muscles need strengthening exercises to prevent back pain. Caution: If you have ever experienced back pain, check with your doctor before you begin these tests.

For the first three movements, lie flat on the floor with your legs straight and your hands behind your neck. Keeping your knees locked, raise both legs 10 inches above the floor and hold for 10 seconds. Next, while a helper holds your feet down, roll up to a sitting position. Finally, roll back down, bend your knees to bring them as close as possible to your chest and do a second sit-up. These movements test the strength of stomach and hip muscles.

Begin the next three movements lying on your stomach with a pillow under your abdomen, while your helper presses one hand on the small of your back and the other on your ankles. Clasping your hands behind your neck, raise your trunk and hold it steady for 10 seconds. Next, still lying prone, fold both arms under your head and lift your legs,

keeping them raised for 10 seconds. Finally, stand up straight with your feet together, gently bend over, and try to touch the floor, keeping knees straight. These final movements gauge the strength and flexibility of the muscles around the spine.

Why a back goes out of whack

Despite all tests and precautions, the back is predisposed to occasional breakdown and, given its intricate structure, it is easy to see why. Even a minor mechanical failure can lead to agony, because within the spine lies the center of a complex network of branching nerves, which send a distress signal of pain if any of the spine's components is damaged or diseased.

The crucial components are 24 movable bones, the vertebrae, running from the skull to the pelvis. Seven of them, in the neck, support the head; 12 in the chest anchor the ribs; five at the small of the back bear the weight of the upper body (Chapter 1). Each consists of a solid cylinder and an attached hollow ring; the rings line up to form the spinal canal, which

The weighty job of the spine

The reason back injuries are so common has been demonstrated by the research of Swedish physician Dr. Alf Nachemson and research engineer Gosta Elfström. They implanted a tiny measuring device in the third lumbar disc of a healthy young woman and recorded the pressures created by various postures and physical activities (right), some performed with a 22-pound weight in each hand. They found that coughing places the lower spine under pressures greater than those generated in the cylinders of a small automobile engine. And doing sit-ups creates bone-crushing stresses equal to the pressure on a submarine hull 570 feet down.

Lifting 44 pounds improperly—with back bent and knees locked—places almost twice as much stress on the lumbar disc as performing the same task properly, with knees bent and back straight. Likewise, bending forward 30 degrees or more causes twice as much lumbar pressure as standing straight. But leaning forward while sitting—a position often assumed by drivers and desk-bound workers—is even more stressful than bending forward while standing. Even laughter can be dangerous; the sudden jolting of the entire body during a fit of giggles places more pressure on the lumbar area than jumping up and down.

protects the nerves of the spinal cord. Bony outgrowths—long "processes" and, between them, rounded "facets"—jut from each ring; you can feel the processes that project toward the rear by running a finger along the spine.

Processes serve as anchors for muscles; the facets help keep the spine from bending excessively. It bends as much and as smoothly as it does because of two sets of joints. One is made up of cushions of connective tissue, called discs, lying between the vertebrae's solid cylinders. A capsule of soft gelatinous material, each disc functions somewhat like a shock absorber, shifting its contents to absorb the body's jolts and twists; the outer wall of a disc is made up of layers of ligaments, crisscrossed like the plies in a radial tire, to make a firm connection between two vertebrae. The second set of joints consists of flexible connections between the facets, which line up along both sides of the spine.

Below the movable sections of the spine lie two groups of vertebrae. Five vertebrae form the rear of the pelvis; another

four—collectively called the coccyx—anchor the rectal area. Unless they are fractured by a accident, neither group of vertebrae is likely back pain. Another relatively safe area is the between the rear of the pelvis and the two f the notion that backache could be blamed a fallacy. But a real battle zone of the b where the endlessly moving vertebrae in meet the unyielding ones in the pelvis

Every day the small of the back und near-violent stress. Leaning down an weight—the weight of a five-year the lower back of an adult to more sure per square inch if done wrong— legs and back bent at the waist. The rigia ab-sorb the force of the thrust; instead, the five v above and their joints take the brunt of it. The number and kinds of injuries that can result from such stress are awesome;

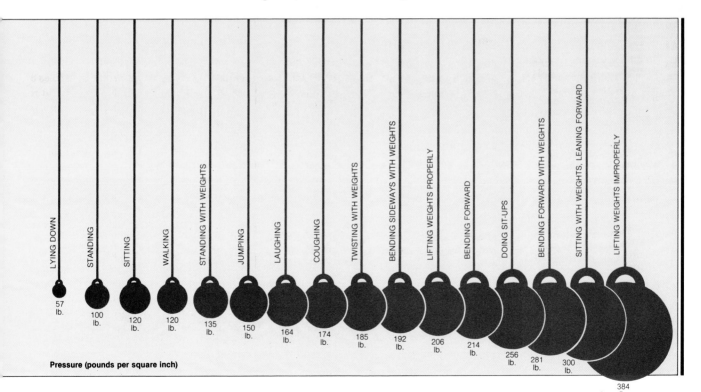

Pressure (pounds per square inch)

Activity	Pressure
LYING DOWN	57 lb.
STANDING	100 lb.
SITTING	120 lb.
WALKING	120 lb.
STANDING WITH WEIGHTS	135 lb.
JUMPING	150 lb.
LAUGHING	164 lb.
COUGHING	174 lb.
TWISTING WITH WEIGHTS	185 lb.
BENDING SIDEWAYS WITH WEIGHTS	192 lb.
LIFTING WEIGHTS PROPERLY	206 lb.
BENDING FORWARD	214 lb.
DOING SIT-UPS	256 lb.
BENDING FORWARD WITH WEIGHTS	281 lb.
SITTING WITH WEIGHTS, LEANING FORWARD	300 lb.
LIFTING WEIGHTS IMPROPERLY	384 lb.

one medical text lists 103 separate causes of low-back pain.

But a Columbia and New York University study of 5,000 back patients found that some 80 per cent of all backaches arise from one source: injured muscles and ligaments. Long before the pangs of this type of injury are felt in the spine itself, a victim is likely to feel muscle pain in the general area of the lower back, particularly when the muscles are fatigued. Among these critical muscles are those of the abdomen, which help hold the trunk erect. If the abdominal muscles are weakened by lack of exercise or by being stretched to handle added weight, the other muscles of the back will be called upon for extra duty. In effect, then, trouble in the back is very likely to begin in trouble at the front of the body.

Many backache patients find this concept hard to accept. Orthopedist Lawrence Friedman recalled a burly dock worker who came to him complaining of severe back pain. When Friedman informed him that the cause of his ailment was weak stomach muscles, the dock worker scoffed. ''Doc,'' he said, ''I can lift two of you with each hand.'' While conceding that this might be so, the doctor pointed out that his patient had been unable to do sit-ups during an examination. Dr. Friedman gestured toward the man's diminutive wife and said he was willing to bet that her stomach muscles were stronger for her weight than her husband's. When the dock worker cheerfully agreed to the wager, Dr. Friedman asked the wife to get up on the examining table. As he expected, she was able to do repeated sit-ups. The embarrassed husband dutifully undertook a program of abdomen-strengthening exercises, and his back pain soon disappeared.

Compounding the problems of weak abdominal muscles is one of its visible results: a protruding belly. The belly pulls the lower back forward. To compensate, the buttocks tend to project backward. Together, these two distortions exaggerate the curve in the small of the back, creating a swayback called lordosis. Lordosis not only distorts the spine, putting extra stress on the hard-working discs, but it puts a permanent strain on the muscles around the lower back.

Subjected to a very severe stress, the muscles or ligaments may actually tear, causing instant and acute pain. Often, however, worse is yet to come—an attack of muscle spasm.

Nearby muscles go into contraction, partly to defend themselves against tearing, partly to act as a kind of rigid splint for the injury, guarding it against further movement. The response is one of the body's most valuable safety mechanisms, but it usually produces excruciating pain, often more severe and always more widespread than that of the original injury. A back in spasm locks up, virtually immobilizing the entire body. The only remedy is to try to relax and wait for the spasm to subside—as it generally will. Eventually the muscle or ligament will also heal, though it may be more susceptible to tearing if subjected to another overload.

Spasm can also be caused by emotional stress and muscular tension. The most familiar result of muscle tightness is the so-called tension headache, but people prone to anxiety or unable to work off frustrations by physical means may find their back muscles tensing as well.

Dr. John V. Basmajian, of McMaster University in Ontario, Canada, described this emotionally caused type of backache as ''a tension headache that has slipped down the back.'' The affliction is widespread—some experts believe that as many as 80 per cent of all backaches are caused by psychological stress—and a spasm brought on by tension is every bit as excruciating as one brought on by a muscle or ligament injury. ''Most often,'' observed Dr. John Sarno of New York's Institute of Rehabilitative Medicine, ''it's the conscientious, compulsive type of person who is susceptible.'' Thus, office workers who complain, ''The boss is on my back,'' may be speaking the truth.

While injuries or psychological tensions may produce most back pain, their effects are relatively brief; the commonest site of serious back trouble is the discs. Even in perfect condition, the discs show wear and tear. During each day, in younger people they shrink 20 to 30 per cent under the pressure and pounding of routine motion, as moisture seeps out of their cores and through the outer wall; by evening, an average adult is about half an inch shorter than when arising.

During a night's sleep, the discs reabsorb moisture and regain their size and bounce, but over the course of a lifetime, beginning about age 20, they dry out slightly, and gradually undergo a permanent compression. Older people actually do

An engineering analysis of stresses and strains

Doctors who treat backaches confess that much of what they do is guesswork. No one knows how to cure all the aches because no one knows precisely how the spine and its guying muscles work, let alone how and why they malfunction to cause pain. To find answers to these questions, researchers have put volunteers through a variety of experiments. The subjects pull, push or twist while detectors taped to their trunks pick up the electrical signals that indicate how hard a given muscle is working.

So far the conclusions are basic—confirming, for example, the common knowledge that a weight held close to the body causes less strain than the same weight held with arms outstretched. Yet this research also quantifies the difference: An 18-pound weight held at arm's length strains the back twice as much as if held close. "We are just beginning to gather the needed information," said Dr. Albert Schultz, Director of the University of Illinois Biomechanics Research Laboratory, "but the more we can learn about the mechanical behavior of the back, the better we can contribute to prevention, diagnosis and treatment of its problems."

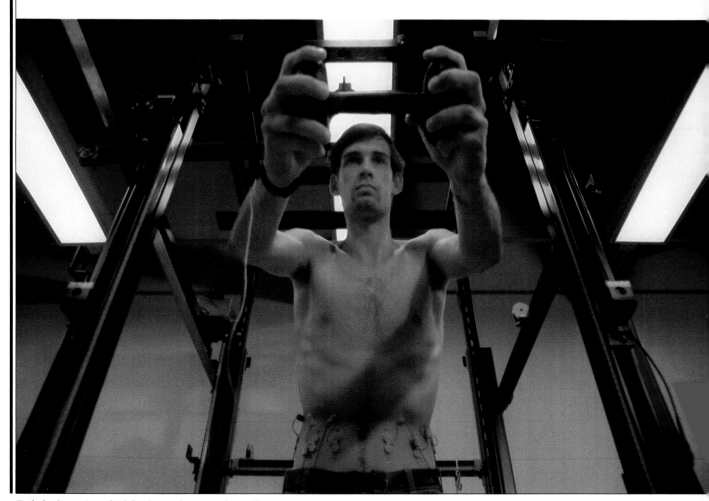

To help determine which back muscles control specific movements, a volunteer at the University of Illinois lab raises and lowers an 11-pound bar bell while electrodes pasted to his waist sense the nerve impulses that make muscles contract. The experiment indicated that lifting and lowering involve all the muscles that run along either side of the backbone.

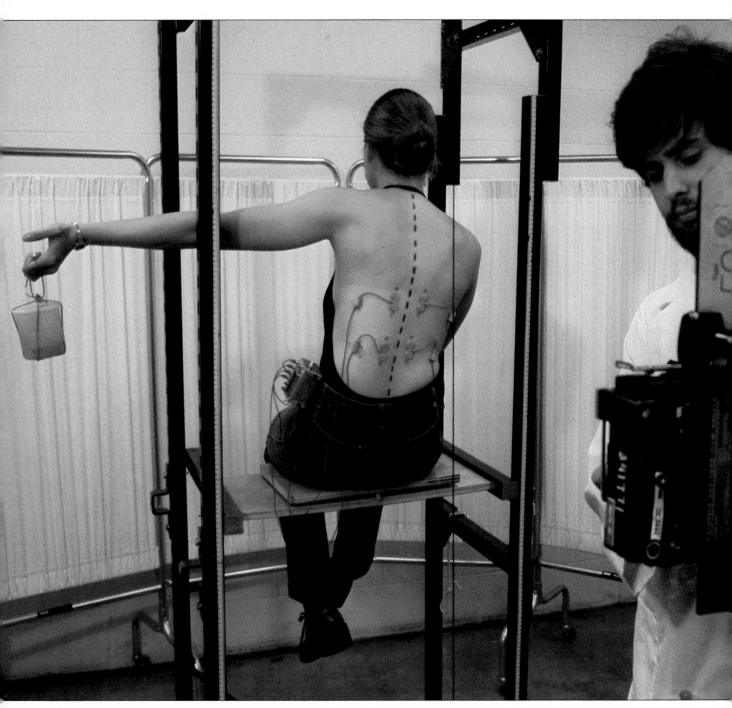

The effect on the back of a 3½-pound weight held at arm's length is gauged by photographing the deviation of the subject's spine, marked with dye, from the thin black plumb line hanging down the frame. Electrodes taped to her back measure muscle action, and calibrations on the frame reveal weight shifts.

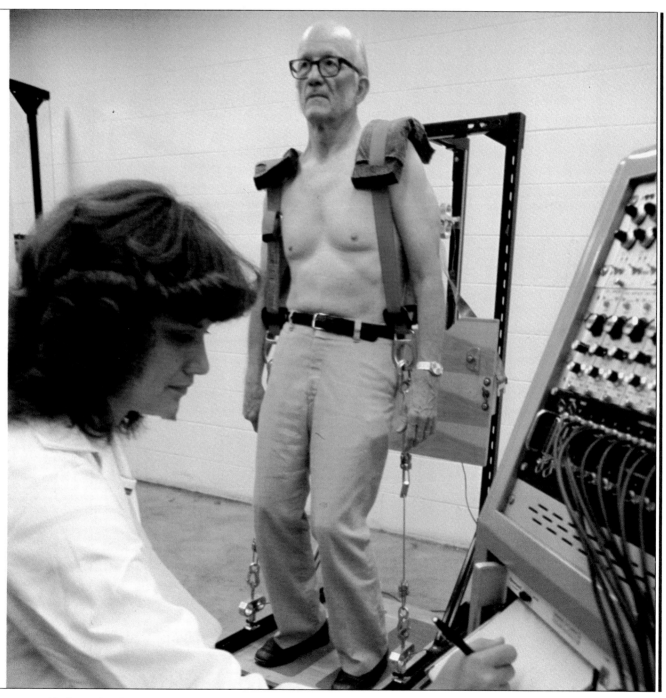

A man with chronic low-back pain presses up on a shoulder harness wired to a machine that measures the force of the thrust. The test is designed to see how different kinds and levels of pressure aggravate back conditions—information that someday may help doctors predict and prevent painful attacks.

become shorter as the years pass. The passing years may also bring more serious consequences. Inevitably a disc wall begins to weaken, and many tiny tears may develop in the outer wall. In its weakened state, a disc under stress may suddenly give way, creating the condition called a slipped disc.

The term is misleading: A disc does not actually slip or shift out of position; it undergoes a partial collapse. Generally, a section of the outer wall thins and bulges out like a weak spot on a tire. Occasionally, the outer wall breaks and some of the pulpy core bursts completely out of the disc.

A protruding or ruptured disc can cause pain in several ways. The damaged disc occupies less space, and nearby muscles work overtime—and may go into spasm—as they struggle to keep the vertebrae aligned. Second, the body's protective system may attack loose bits of extruded pulp as if they were disease-causing invaders, producing inflammation and swelling in surrounding tissues. Finally, and most crucially, the bulging outer wall or extruded pulp may press on one of the nerve roots that branch out from the spinal cord.

Not surprisingly, the disc most frequently injured is the one that bears the most pressure—the lowest movable disc in the small of the back just above the pelvis. The likeliest outcome of such a rupture is a searing pain on one or both sides, radiating down the outer side of the buttock and thigh, over the front of the knee, down the inner side of the leg toward the big toe. Other damaged discs may produce pain in the hip, the thigh or the side. The pain of these lower-back ailments generally increases when the spine is bent forward.

The pain caused by discs is most common in the middle years. The back heals itself with age, for as the discs shrink, the spine produces bone projections—spurs—and the facets reshape themselves. This restructuring helps to stabilize the discs so that they cannot protrude and it also provides extra room for the nerves. As the back continues to stiffen with advancing years, it becomes less flexible; with less bending and twisting of the spine there is less pain from the discs.

A ruptured disc also causes pain in the small of the back. However, low-back pain can also signal any of several facet-joint ailments, collectively called the facet-joint syndrome. In every case, a compressed disc lets the facets grind against each other, irritating tiny nerves and ultimately destroying the cartilage between them. Sometimes the facets produce bony spurs that touch nearby nerves; or nearby nerves may be irritated when facet joints are dislocated slightly by a sudden twist or blow. Generally, a worn or dislocated joint will be most painful when the spine is arched backward.

A number of other ailments can cause pain similar to that of a broken disc or faulty facet joint. Hairline fractures of vertebrae caused by sudden compression, as in a fall, inevitably produce pain. So do tumors in the spinal canal, and infections of membranes that sheathe the spinal nerves. Sciatica is a sharp pain caused by inflammation of the two sciatic nerves, which run from the lower back, across the buttocks and down the thighs; the inflammation is sometimes produced by a muscle spasm pressing on either of these nerves.

The litany of back pain includes a list of ills that are not directly associated with the back but cause pain there. The messages that run through the spinal cord are sometimes hard for the brain to disentangle. Ulcers, malfunctioning kidneys, an ailing prostate, even a sick heart, in sending their distress signals to the brain by way of the cord, can trigger backache. Referred pain, as such neurological short circuits are termed, makes backache diagnosis tricky even for the experts.

Fortunately, most low-back pain involves nothing more than muscle fatigue and spasm; even the disorders of discs and facet joints are likely to affect the muscles, and most doctors wait for the muscle spasm to subside before trying to treat the underlying cause. Almost invariably, a pain that requires immediate medical attention is accompanied by nonmuscular symptoms. Persistent numbness or tingling, for example, may signal nerve damage. Other danger signs include fever, urinary or bowel difficulties, stomach disorders or menstrual irregularities. Backache after an injury, or pain so severe that it prevents sleep are still other causes for concern—and for immediate medical attention.

What to do when backache strikes

In the absence of nonmuscular symptoms, you can assume that—for the moment, at least—you can deal with back pain yourself. First take a painkiller such as aspirin or acetaminophen. Then go to bed and stay there—almost any doctor will recommend this course, whatever your difficulty. In an upright position, your back muscles work strenuously simply to keep you erect; lying down relieves them of that task, helps them to relax their self-defensive spasm, and reduces the chances of aggravating an injury.

Lie on a firm surface that holds your spine steady. Though a pliable, yielding mattress is acceptable for ordinary bed rest, any movement can cause anguish during a backache. Many victims are most comfortable lying on a carpeted floor; some prefer a mattress placed on the floor. Lie in a position that straightens your spine—either on your back with a small pillow under your head and a larger one beneath your knees, or on your side with your legs tucked up and your head on a pillow just large enough to keep your back straight. During a particularly acute spasm, you may find that lying on the floor with your feet on a chair is the most comfortable position. Do not lie on your stomach—it accentuates your spinal curvature and will heighten your suffering.

Stay flat in bed, even for meals if possible. If you must rise to a sitting position, try to have someone help you. To get out of bed with the aid of a helper, lie on your side, ease your legs over the edge of the bed and gradually rise to a sitting position; then, leaning on your helper for support, stand up slowly. If you are alone, roll onto all fours across the bed, crawl backward and reach down to the floor one leg at a time. If your bed has a headboard, use it to steady yourself as you rise. Reverse the procedure to return to bed.

To soothe your muscles and speed the relaxing of a spasm, apply either heat or cold to the area of pain. The two work in different ways; most doctors agree that your choice should depend primarily on what feels best to you. Most people find heat more effective. It relaxes muscles and speeds the flow of blood into the area (the increased blood supply aids the repair of torn muscles). Use a heating pad at a low setting, a heat lamp or a hot-water bottle; if you prefer a moist heat, use a warm wet towel or a heat pack called a hydrocollator, available at pharmacies, which retains the heat of boiling water. Do not apply heat for more than 15 minutes at a time.

Cold, while less soothing, works well in reducing particu-larly severe pain. It numbs tissues, and it reduces inflammation by constricting blood vessels; eventually the exhausted muscles begin to relax. Cold can be applied with an ice pack; if you do not have one, place some ice cubes in a plastic bag and rub them over the painful area.

Massage also helps. Lie on your stomach with a pillow under your abdomen to keep your back straight. You do not need a professional masseur. Have a companion massage your back with the heels of the hands, using gentle pressure in a kneading motion, starting at the buttocks and working upward and outward from the spinal column.

After a few days, or whenever your back is no longer locked in spasm and your pain has diminished somewhat, start moving a bit in bed, stretching your arms and legs and shifting your position from time to time. When the pain abates further, start a few simple exercises, such as tightening your abdominal muscles and rotating your pelvis to flatten your spine against the bed. These movements are a foretaste of the rehabilitation exercises that will come later, and the sooner you get started on them, the better off you will be. But be cautious: If any movement proves painful, abandon it until you feel stronger.

The same cautions apply to sexual activity. It is temporarily out of the question for anyone experiencing acute back pain, and many backache victims avoid intercourse long after they have recovered from the acute stage, out of fear that it will trigger another attack. In reality, once the pain has subsided there is no reason not to resume sexual relations. Most physicians agree that the basic pelvic movements of conventional intercourse are a good therapy for an ailing back.

Once you are on your feet again and able to walk without pain—usually within five to seven days—start exercising your back every day. Exercises like those on pages 64 and 65 limber and strengthen the muscles around the lower spine, building up a flexible internal brace that can guard your back against further injuries. But the key to lasting health is a routine of regular, continuing exercise. Dr. Leon Root, of New York City's Hospital for Special Surgery, once pointed out that an injured back is never completely cured. "Low-back pain," he said, "is your warning that something is

What really happens when a disc "slips"

The human spine is akin to a perilously balanced stack of poker chips: Intricately sculpted interlocking bones, called vertebrae, are cushioned by resilient discs, lashed together with sturdy ligaments and guyed upright by a host of muscles. In a normal, healthy back, the discs, which have the consistency of stale gumdrops, act as miniature shock absorbers, and pairs of small vertebral projections called facets line up, one above the other, to create smoothly functioning joints.

Both the discs and the facet joints show the effects of steady use as the years go by. The discs dry out somewhat and lose a degree of resiliency; the facet joints begin to wear. In people suffering from severe back pain, the process has generally been exaggerated—by disease that speeds up the degeneration, by the trauma of injury or, most commonly, by the stresses that the spine must bear if there is insufficient muscular support. The result may be either what is commonly but incorrectly known as a slipped disc—a disc that has partially collapsed or ruptured under pressure—or painfully grinding facet joints.

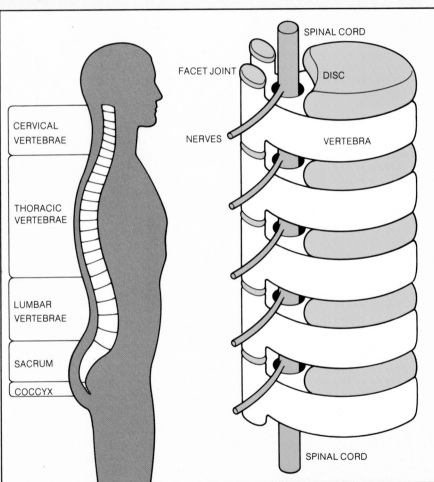

THE SPRINGY SPINE'S CURVE
Stacked in an S curve that gives flexibility, the spine has five sections. The jointed neck (cervical), chest (thoracic) and lower-back (lumbar) regions have 24 individual vertebrae; fused, unmovable groups form the pelvic area (sacrum) and tail (coccyx).

BUILDING BLOCKS OF THE BACK
Between the skull and pelvis, the spine consists of movable vertebrae, separated by discs in the front and connected at facet joints in the rear. Through a hole in each vertebra runs the spinal cord, sprouting nerves that lead to other parts of the body.

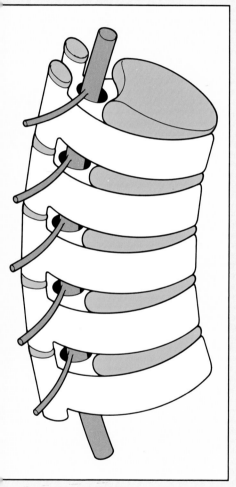

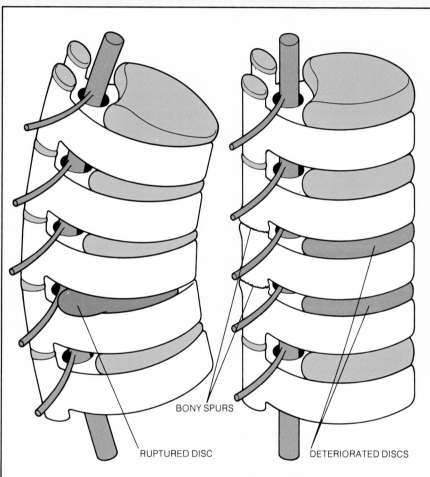

BONY SPURS

RUPTURED DISC

DETERIORATED DISCS

HOW DISCS ABSORB SHOCKS

When the back is bent forward (above), the front of each disc compresses and the rear expands. The disc contracts at the rear if the spine is bent backward. In a healthy back, the disc springs back to its natural shape when the spine straightens again.

THE RUPTURED OR "SLIPPED" DISC

A weak spot in ligaments encasing it lets the disc bulge out; the bulge presses on a nerve and induces the radiating pain of a so-called slipped disc. Eventually, the casing may break, spilling the gel-like nucleus of the disc and compounding the pain.

FAULTY FACET JOINTS

When a disc deteriorates and flattens permanently, the space between vertebrae narrows. The facets abrade each other, wear down cartilage and produce bony spurs that touch nearby nerves. A twisting injury can yield similar results.

wrong. The next time it hits it will be worse. What you have to do is heed this warning and take steps to prevent the problem from ever occurring again.'' The most important single step, orthopedists agree, is a lifelong commitment to daily exercise.

Failure to exercise inevitably invites another attack. Paul Hendricks, a Philadelphia businessman who injured his back while swinging one of his children in the air, exercised religiously for a year and a half. Then, supposing that the trouble had cleared up, he tapered off. One day, while driving to work, he stopped for a traffic light and reached back to the rear seat for his newspaper. A newsmagazine account of the incident described what happened next: ''The light changed, horns honked, traffic moved. Not Hendricks.'' His back had gone into spasm. A state trooper spent half an hour getting him out of his car. After three weeks of bed rest and intensive treatment, Hendricks went back to his exercises.

Medical solutions for persistent pain

Though the ultimate responsibility in caring for a bad back falls mainly to the victim, anyone with acute pain or with persistent, recurring backaches needs professional help.

The diagnosis for a persistent backache is an intricate exercise in medical detection. To gather clues, doctors observe how a patient walks, stands, bends and climbs onto the examining table. They may take precise measurements to see if one leg is significantly shorter or one shoulder lower than the other. The reactions to such standard and familiar reflex tests as tapping the knee joints with a small rubber hammer get close scrutiny, and so do the responses to pinpricks in the affected area: Both yield clues about affected nerves.

The solution to a backache mystery can spring from apparently trivial gleanings. One man crippled by lower-back pain could offer no information to reveal the cause of his condition. Finally the doctor asked him if he carried a briefcase to work. Yes, he did. Was it usually heavy, inquired the doctor. ''Very,'' was the reply. And with which hand, the doctor pursued, did he carry it? ''Well, I've always carried it with my right hand,'' said the patient, ''but a couple of weeks ago I changed over and began carrying it with my left hand.''

Suddenly the answer was obvious: The man had wrenched his back by the abrupt and continuing shift in load.

Another man complained that he had been troubled for more than a year by sciatica. After some discussion the doctor happened to notice that his patient carried a wallet crammed with credit cards in his hip pocket. The thick wad of leather and plastic pressed a point directly above the sciatic nerve. The doctor simply recommended moving the wallet to another pocket and the patient soon recovered.

Most back problems are not resolved that easily. If preliminary probings do not solve the puzzle, a doctor will make an X-ray picture to see the positioning of the vertebrae. Ordinary X-rays, however, have their limitations: Though they clearly show curvatures, twists and some misalignments of the spine, they pick up no more than a vague indication of the soft discs between the vertebrae. If a ruptured disc is the suspected source of trouble, the doctor may order a myelogram, for which a dye opaque to X-rays is injected into the spinal canal before the picture is made. The patient is placed on a table and the dye is injected into the lower spinal canal, below the end of the spinal cord so that the needle will not damage the cord; then the table is tilted, the dye flows up the spinal canal and the X-rays are taken. In the finished picture, the spinal cavity shows up as a dense white column in which the bulge from any rupture makes a distinct indentation.

To see the intricate facet joints that flank the spine, a physician may turn to an even more sophisticated X-ray technique: computerized axial tomography, which produces the so-called CAT scan. An X-ray source circles around the patient's midriff, taking progressively deeper concentric views, and a computer converts all the shots into one detailed cross-section picture. The procedure is expensive, but it is the best way to detect and diagnose facet-joint problems.

Muscular abnormalities do not show up on any X-ray, but they can be studied in an electromyogram, a picture of electrical activity. A contracting muscle generates electrical impulses; the more it is tensed, the more impulses it produces. To make an electromyogram, fine needles are inserted into the back to pick up these electrical impulses, which are converted into sound and also into a pattern on a screen. The

Who hurts his back and why

Low-back pain is the most common occupational complaint, afflicting one of every two American workers at least once during their careers. Back injuries cost American industry an estimated $14 billion annually.

Workers whose jobs require heavy lifting, pulling, pushing or carrying, such as miners, lumbermen and warehousemen, understandably suffer the most in terms of workdays lost *(below)*. But truck drivers, who spend most of their workdays sitting, are also particularly vulnerable, probably because lack of proper support

for the lower back in driving seats, coupled with continuous vibration, takes a toll on the fourth and fifth discs of the lower back.

Restaurant workers, who like warehousemen bend and lift, lose little time to back injuries; most are young and physically fit, and their loads are relatively light and within easy reach on table tops or counters. But doctors, nurses and others who care for the sick are nearly as vulnerable as construction workers. Lifting and moving patients is as stressful to the lower back as hefting building materials.

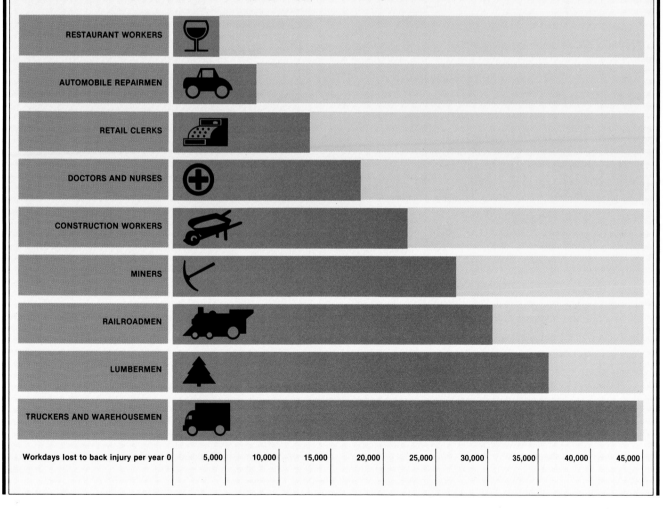

RESTAURANT WORKERS									
AUTOMOBILE REPAIRMEN									
RETAIL CLERKS									
DOCTORS AND NURSES									
CONSTRUCTION WORKERS									
MINERS									
RAILROADMEN									
LUMBERMEN									
TRUCKERS AND WAREHOUSEMEN									

Workdays lost to back injury per year   0   5,000   10,000   15,000   20,000   25,000   30,000   35,000   40,000   45,000

sound and the visible pattern can reveal muscular abnormalities and certain diseases of the spine itself.

After assembling and weighing all of the clues, most physicians start with a conservative prescription: bed rest, sometimes in a hospital.

For a ruptured disc, the classic treatment has included traction, in which a girdle around the pelvis is attached to 15-to-30-pound weights slung over the edge of the bed; in a somewhat less common method, the patient is suspended from the shoulders on a tilted bed or platform. In theory, artificial weights or the weight of the patient's body gently pull the spine to increase the spaces between vertebrae, relieving any pressure of a disc upon a nerve. Most back patients find their pain dramatically reduced during a typical 10-to-12-day course of treatment. Nevertheless, traction is increasingly a subject of controversy among doctors. In a Norwegian study, several hundred back patients were placed in conventional traction harnesses, but weights were installed on only half of them. There was no difference in the rate of recovery between the two groups.

Such experiments have led many doctors to argue that the value of traction lies not in the weights but in the fact that the patient is literally tied down while the back heals itself. Dr. George Hyatt, Chief of Orthopedics at Georgetown University Hospital, made a forceful statement of that hospital's general position. "Most back problems will correct themselves within three weeks, no matter what we do," he said. The object of most conventional medical remedies for back pain, then, is to keep the patient as still and comfortable as possible while the body's healing forces do their work.

Part of making patients comfortable is the temporary use of pain-relieving drugs. If aspirin proves ineffective, a doctor will prescribe a somewhat stronger but nonnarcotic painkiller such as propoxyphene or pentazocine. For severe pain, he may prescribe morphine or a synthetic equivalent, but for only a brief period because of the danger of addiction. Tranquilizers help patients if emotional tension has led to muscle spasm; muscle relaxants break the pain-spasm-pain cycle, in which muscle pain produces a spasm, and the spasm irritates nerves, provoking further pain and spasm. Some doctors inject drugs directly into the back; a common concoction combines a local anesthetic with anti-inflammation drugs.

Like the home therapist, doctors also have drugless methods for reducing pain. One is heat, often induced by microwave diathermy. A diathermy machine works rather like a microwave oven, producing a rapidly alternating electrical field that agitates molecules in the tissues. Cold can be applied in the form of ethyl chloride, the same substance that television viewers sometimes see athletic trainers spraying on players' injured limbs as an anesthetic. Or a physician may try a counterirritant, such as a cream or liquid containing methyl salicylate or oil of wintergreen, which, like the old-fashioned mustard plaster, irritates the skin and stimulates underlying nerves; when the technique works, it is because the nerves have increased the activity of nearby muscles so that they go out of spasm.

Once the worst of the pain is gone, a doctor often refers the patient to a physical therapist, who may apply further heat or cold treatments, administer massages and devise a rehabilitative exercise program. During this transition period, the doctor may advise the temporary use of a brace or a therapeutic corset. Braces immobilize the spine; they are generally prescribed for people with seriously injured backs. Some types, however, correct inborn abnormalities such as a sideways curvature of the spine; these are often used on growing children. Corsets are essentially strong, elastic sashes that provide support for weak muscles in the back and abdomen.

Ready-made braces and corsets, widely available at drugstores and other commercial outlets, are sometimes advertised as backache cures. They are nothing of the kind. Such a device should not be used unless a doctor has prescribed it and a certified fitter has measured the patient for it. Ill-fitting braces can do more harm than good, and over a long period of time corsets actually weaken the very muscles that need strengthening to provide inner support for the back.

When all else fails—surgery
Despite all of the therapies and gadgetry, the time may come when an operation offers the only means of permanent relief. Continued but moderate discomfort is not in itself a sufficient

reason for surgery; Dr. Bernard Tinneson of Hahnemann Medical College in Philadelphia observed, "If you can cope with the pain, you don't need surgery," adding that in the confines of the spinal canal the scars of an operation can produce as much discomfort as the condition the operation was meant to correct.

Therefore, surgery is generally restricted to such problems as a severe fracture of the spine, a tumor or a threat to nerves or organs, and to pain that is still too severe to be tolerated after all other means of relief have been tried. Such cases are relatively rare. According to Dr. C. Norman Shealy, Director of the Pain and Health Rehabilitation Center in La Crosse, Wisconsin, "Probably in not more than one per cent of patients with fairly severe back pain is surgery ever indicated." Shealy, like most orthopedists, made it a habit to urge patients to get a second opinion before agreeing to surgery. Said a New York orthopedist, Dr. John Doherty, "If my recommendation has been based not so much on ironclad evidence like X-rays, as on my own hunch based on experience, I will even suggest the names of other physicians that might be consulted." Both Drs. Shealy and Doherty emphasized that a patient should proceed only if both doctors agree; if they disagree, a third opinion is in order.

Of all spinal operations, by far the most common is a laminectomy, designed to correct a broken disc. To reach the disc, the surgeon makes an opening in the lamina, a wall-like section of bone at the back of the vertebra. Past this barrier, he gently moves the spinal nerve roots aside, inspects the damaged disc and removes any part of the whitish, pulpy core that presses against a nerve root; if the disc is greatly deteriorated, he may reach inside and scrape out all of the core. Aside from the obvious dangers involved in working so close to the spinal nerves—an accidental nick can cause paralysis—a laminectomy is an uncomplicated procedure. Said Dr. Sam Wiesel, an orthopedic surgeon at George Washington University Hospital, "The most difficult problem is making the decision to operate."

In discussions with his patients, Wiesel was blunt about the risks. Said one patient, Homer Lange: "He told me, 'I can kill you, I can cripple you for life or I can give you a severe infection.' " For Lange, a Washington, D.C., businessman whom Wiesel described as a "classic disc case," the risks were worth it. A physically active man in his early 40s, Lange had a long history of low-back pain. "I stupidly ignored all the signs," he said. But at Christmastime in 1980 he picked up a load of firewood and a pain shot down his left leg—a pain far too severe to ignore. A Christian Scientist, Lange customarily refused all drugs, but when he checked into the hospital in early April, he was, he said, "living on painkillers."

When he woke up from the anesthetic, the searing sciatica that had plagued him for months was completely gone. The day after the operation he was up on his feet. By the time he left the hospital, seven days after surgery, the temporary discomfort caused by swelling—"It felt like I was lying on a baseball"—had disappeared, and within a month he was walking three to four miles a day.

The complete success of Lange's operation fitted the usual pattern of a laminectomy. Few patients ever need the second-most-common type of back operation, a spinal fusion, which stabilizes the area from which disc material has been partially or completely removed. A fusion is essentially a bone graft. The surgeon scrapes away the surface of the two unstable vertebrae, using instruments that look like miniature cabinet-making tools. Elsewhere in the body—a favorite site is the pelvis—he chisels out a number of matchstick-like slivers of soft inner bone. The surgeon uses the bits of bone to assemble a sort of trellis connecting the two vertebrae; this structure serves as a base on which the body grows new bone, eventually fusing the vertebrae into a single strong unit.

Back magic: the alternative treatments

For a surprisingly large group of backache victims, neither traditional conservative treatments nor surgery brings relief. Some suffer severe pain, but no injury or illness can be detected; others have something physically awry that either is not serious enough for surgery or has already been operated on without success. Such victims of chronic backache often seek relief in an array of therapies offered by practitioners on the fringes of the conventional medical establishment.

Some of these alternative treatments have no recognized medical value; others are innovative or speculative techniques that are not completely proved but are undergoing serious scientific investigation.

One of the oldest of the nonconventional treatments is spinal manipulation, a technique for pushing supposedly misaligned vertebrae back into position by manual pressure. Sufferers from mild spinal curvatures or facet-joint ailments have found relief in the method, but most doctors, even those who sometimes practice the technique themselves, point out that it is not likely to have permanent results; within days the spine resumes its previous contours. What is more, the procedure can be dangerous in unskilled hands. Spinal-cord damage caused by manipulation, generally in the delicate neck vertebrae, has brought on paralysis or even death. According to one orthopedist, the best way to guard against such dangers is to ask a physician to suggest a qualified practitioner—"and then don't let him work on your neck."

Most trained spinal manipulators are either osteopaths or chiropractors. The two groups share similar theories and are often linked in the public mind, but there are crucial differences between them.

The founder of osteopathy, a Missouri physician named Andrew Taylor Still, worked out his theories in the 1870s. Dr. Still believed that all human ailments, from measles to cancer, arose from minor spinal dislocations that could be corrected by manipulation. For many years osteopaths clung to this sweeping creed and were regarded as cultists by the medical establishment. But in recent decades their training has been broadened and greatly improved; it is now accepted by the American Medical Association as comparable to that of conventional medical schools. In some parts of the United States, doctors of osteopathy, or D.O.s, are permitted to take the same state licensing examinations as M.D.s. In addition they may prescribe drugs, perform surgery and practice such specialties as dermatology and obstetrics; many serve as staff physicians in large hospitals. Some use little or no manipulation, and generally those who do use it consider it an adjunct to conventional therapies.

Chiropractic was founded in 1895 by an Iowa grocer named Daniel Palmer, who reportedly cured a janitor's deafness by "adjusting" his spine. From his observations Palmer concluded that all disease can be traced to malfunctions of the nervous system, malfunctions always curable by spinal manipulation. Many modern chiropractors still adhere to this theory; the modern medical establishment rejects it. And though chiropractors now receive a rudimentary medical training, they are forbidden to prescribe drugs and may not perform surgery except in the state of Oregon, where limited minor surgery is permitted.

For the patient, the critical distinctions between the two types of practice are partly a matter of scope, partly a matter of safety. Osteopathic physicians are versed in many medical techniques; chiropractors are limited to one. More important, only the osteopath has the training to identify complex problems that may not respond to manipulation—or that may be intensified by it.

Controversy over a papaya extract

At an opposite extreme from physical manipulation lie drug therapies. One of the most publicized and controversial methods for treating spinal ills is based on a drug called chymopapain, one of the natural substances, known as enzymes, that initiate or accelerate the processes of the body. Derived from the papaya tree, chymopapain is similar to the active ingredient in meat tenderizers. When it is injected into a ruptured disc, the enzyme is supposed to dissolve the pulpy core without harming the surrounding wall; theoretically, the painful disc problem is then resolved without the complications of surgery.

During a decade of clinical trials beginning in the early 1960s, chymopapain showed results ranging from complete relief to no change at all. In 1975 the U.S. Food and Drug Administration ordered investigators to limit injections to well-controlled studies. After this restriction took effect, many Americans received the injections in Canada, and the debate over chymopapain went on. Some doctors warned against the side effects of the drug, including intense allergic reactions, shock and a spasmodic response that closes the larynx and cuts off breathing; two patients are known to have

The controversial practices of chiropractors

Chiropractic, the unorthodox healing art that treats back disorders by pressing and manipulating the spine, has excited controversy since 1895, when its founder, Iowa merchant D. D. Palmer, allegedly restored hearing to a deaf man by forcing a misaligned neck vertebra back into place. Modern Doctors of Chiropractic—there are about 21,000 in the United States—claim no such cures for their technique. Yet they do maintain that the traditional chiropractic methods—sudden thrusts with the hands—can correct certain abnormalities of the spine.

Some practitioners confine their treatment to muscle and bone aches, screening out patients whose pains have other origins. Many, like Drs. James Kalonturos and D. Brent Owens *(right and overleaf),* have added traction, heat therapy and nutritional counseling to the specialized chiropractic procedures.

Even so, the use of chiropractic continues to be challenged. Physicians, while acknowledging that manipulating bones and muscles can relieve some forms of back pain, point out that it can also aggravate existing problems or cause new ones, with complications ranging from heightened pain to nerve damage or stroke. The dangers are increased, physicians believe, by chiropractors' limited diagnostic experience—there is only one chiropractic hospital to provide internships—and by the fact that chiropractors may not prescribe drugs or perform surgery.

Treating a weight lifter for back pain, Dr. Kalonturos uses a precisely aimed, powerful thrust of his right hand, intended to realign a lower-back vertebra. The controversial procedure is accompanied by a characteristic clicking sound.

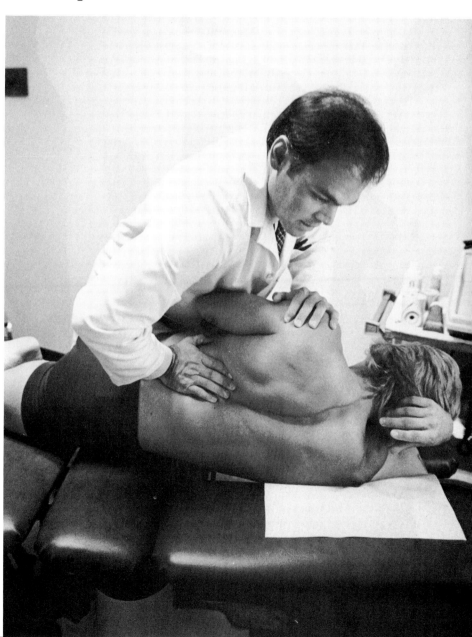

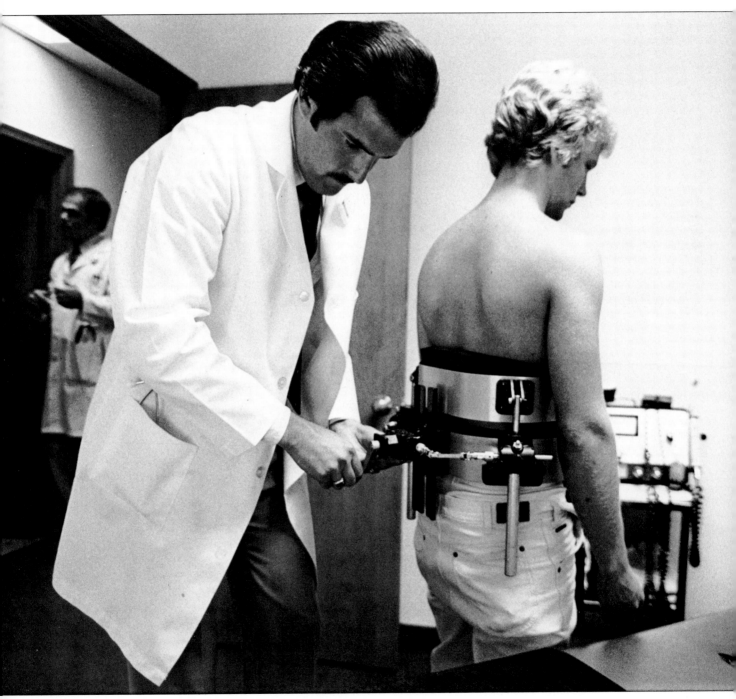

Dr. Owens adjusts the controls on a traction device, consisting of two padded metal bands and a crank, strapped around the lower back of a patient. The device is designed to relieve pain by easing pressure on discs as it forces apart the adjacent vertebrae.

Dr. Kalonturos adjusts the controls on a device chiropractors use for lower-back pain. One harness, strapped around the patient's rib cage, immobilizes the upper body while a second harness, strapped around her waist and fastened to a stationary anchor (not visible), pulls down on her pelvis.

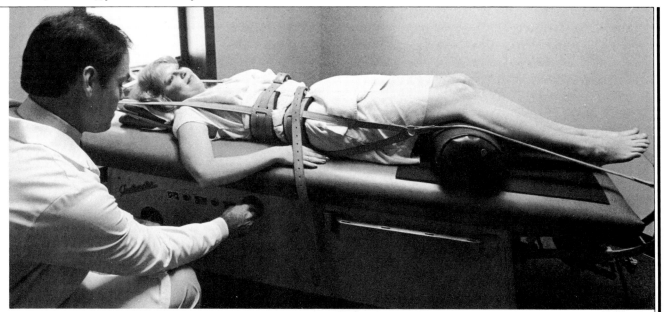

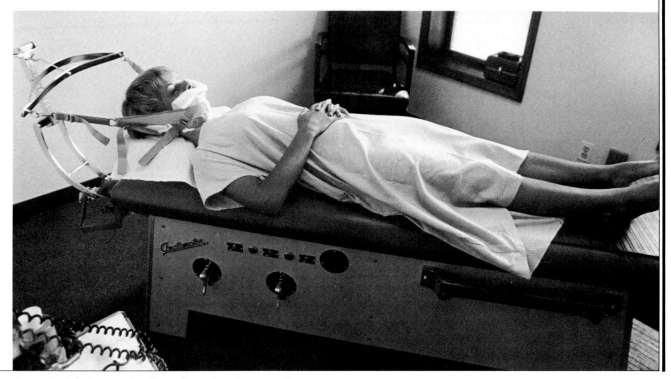

A motorized device stretches the neck muscles of a patient the chiropractor is treating for a muscle spasm. A harness holds the patient's head while the table top—and the patient's lower body—are tugged gently away from the harness every five seconds.

died of such complications. Other doctors feared that the enzyme could leak out of a disc and into surrounding tissue. According to pain expert Dr. Norman Shealy, "Just one drop of the stuff on a capillary and it will hemorrhage."

By contrast, drug treatments called trigger-point injections are generally considered a safe and effective method of treating a special type of back pain, though doctors are at a loss to explain exactly how they work. Trigger points are hard muscular knots, ranging from the size of a pea to the size of a golf ball, and they appear in connective tissue or in muscles that have suffered acute strain or are constantly tense or in spasm. Part of the muscle, in effect, is permanently locked in contraction and apparently develops scarlike adhesions. The result is exquisite pain, and the pain in these areas often provokes, or triggers, further muscle spasm.

To suppress the effect, doctors sometimes inject such trigger points with procaine, a common local anesthetic that numbs the pain in the area and may also unlock the spasm. According to one theory, the injection needle or the pressure of the injected fluid also may break down the adhesions.

The same effect can sometimes be achieved by simply pressing the trigger point with a hard object. When a patient of a New York orthopedist was told that trigger-point injections might allay her severe low-back pain, she expressed fear at being injected. Her doctor persuaded her to let him press the point with the end of a metal cigar container. He applied hard pressure for 10 seconds. The woman screamed —then suddenly cried out, "It doesn't hurt any more!" She stood up and hopped around the room in sheer joy.

The idea of a direct physical attack on trigger points and tensed muscles is also part of certain radical therapies in which the muscles and connective tissue, rather than the joints, are manipulated. Perhaps the most widely known of these techniques is rolfing, named after its founder, American chemist Ida P. Rolf.

Rolfing is not a back treatment as such, but a postural treatment for the entire body. It is sometimes loosely described as a form of massage, though its techniques and effects are markedly different from those of conventional massage. In a series of 10 one-hour sessions, the practitioner, called a rolfer, uses rigid fingers, clenched fists and even elbows to apply pressure to points deep within the body. The pressure is sometimes painful, but in theory it stretches tight muscles and breaks down adhesions on a massive scale, freeing the muscles to guy the spine in its comfortable, upright position. Most physicians regard rolfing as a maverick therapy, but patients who have been successfully rolfed report a dramatically increased flexibility and sense of well-being that often frees them from back pain.

Trigger points figure in the theory of acupuncture, the Chinese healing system based on the idea that pain can be banished by needles inserted at strategic sites on the body. Many of these acupuncture points lie in the areas where trigger points often develop and, like procaine injections, the fine acupuncture needles not only eliminate pain in the immediate area, but banish it from neighboring muscles as well.

But the mechanical effect of the needles on trigger points is only part of the story. An increasing body of evidence suggests that the acupuncture needles also stimulate nerves that signal the brain to release endorphins, natural painkillers secreted by the body.

The release of endorphins may also account for the painkilling effect of electrical devices called transcutaneous nerve stimulators. These machines vary widely in size, from table-top office models, which work through electrodes taped to the ailing back, down to battery-powered models no bigger than a pack of cigarettes, which can be held directly against the skin. Whatever the model, the devices deliver small electric charges to the painful area, and often do relieve pain. Some researchers believe that the electricity stimulates the release of endorphins; others say it overexcites muscles until they become fatigued and loosen their spasm.

Another electrical device sometimes used in back therapy is the biofeedback machine. Like the electromyogram employed for diagnosis, the machine picks up the electrical energy emitted by the contracting muscles. Electrodes on the skin collect the impulses and an amplifier converts the impulses into a signal of light or sound—in effect the machine broadcasts the noise of muscles at work (the sound resembles the ordinary static heard on a radio). Using the device, patients can monitor and often learn to control otherwise involuntary bodily functions such as heart rate, blood pressure, and the spasms of back muscles.

For permanent relief, exercise

Physicians are divided in their opinion of all such unconventional therapies; "Those gimmicks are intriguing, but they are not really in the main line of attack against back problems," said Dr. Doherty. Others take a more guarded view; Dr. B. Berthold Wolff, a pain expert at New York University Medical School, pointed out, "Drugless ways of controlling pain are still considered to be on the oddball fringes of medicine—but they very often work." Even physicians who concede the impressive results of such techniques as acupuncture, transcutaneous nerve stimulation and biofeedback argue that they are limited, because they merely block pain, they do not treat its underlying cause. Most doctors agree that permanent relief from an aching back comes only when patients build up the muscles of the back until it is strong enough to withstand the stresses put on it.

One orthopedist, Lawrence Friedman, recalled a dramatic lesson he received while still in training. One of his distinguished teachers asked for his opinion on some X-rays. What did he think the patient would be capable of doing?

"I looked at the X-rays of the spine," noted Dr. Friedman, "and was horrified. The bones resembled a set of irregular stones; almost all of the intervertebral discs had degenerated. Loose bone fragments could be observed, and there was obviously severe arthritis." Aghast, he said to his teacher that he doubted the person could even walk.

The surgeon smiled and asked the nurse to bring in the patient whose X-rays they were studying. In walked a short, stocky man, moving with a decided bounce. He turned out to be a celebrated Hungarian fencing instructor—and he was in the pink of health. Dr. Friedman subsequently learned that despite periodic attacks of back pain, the man led a thoroughly active life, teaching fencing and even giving lessons in horseback riding to young boys at summer camp. Only his superb muscular conditioning kept him from being a total invalid. But that, it seemed, was enough.   ☀

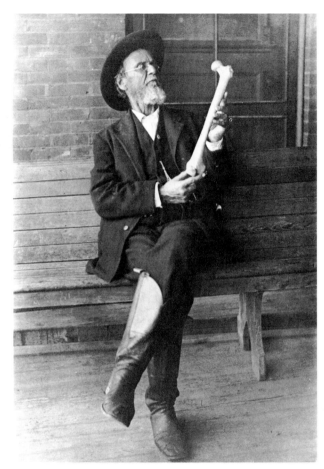

Bespectacled Andrew Taylor Still, the roughhewn frontier doctor who in the mid-19th Century devised the healing system called osteopathy, peers intently at a human thighbone. Still's bone-manipulating treatments, based on his belief that disordered bodily structure could lead to disturbed blood flow and nerve function and thence to disease, brought him ridicule from orthodox practitioners, but many enthusiastic patients. At the time of his death in 1917—at the advanced age of 89—there were more than 5,000 osteopathic physicians in the United States. Almost 19,000 were practicing in the 1980s.

Tricks for avoiding a crick in the spine

The East African tribesmen that Dr. William Kirkaldy-Willis treated during 22 years as a physician in Kenya never rode in cars, sat in chairs or bent over kitchen counters. "They lived the way they have for centuries, and got much more exercise than Westerners," said Dr. Kirkaldy-Willis. "They squatted to work and cook and eat. They always flexed their knees and hips when they bent down. And they all had very good posture." Virtually none complained of a bad back.

Few people in the modern world can avoid trick backs by living the way the East African tribesmen did. Even so their example—frequent exercise, good posture and efficient body mechanics—can help anyone prevent backache. If you properly perform life's commonplace movements—standing, bending, lifting, sitting, reclining (illustrated opposite and on the following pages)—you can eliminate or minimize most of the stresses that can lead to back pain.

These methods of adjusting your body stem from the cardinal rule of good back health: Maintain, as closely as possible, the natural contours of your spine and avoid accentuating its natural, gentle curves (right). For example, every time you bend forward from the waist you curve your back and force your vertebrae to support more than their share of body weight; to counterbalance this stress, you need do nothing more than tilt your pelvis forward to straighten the small of the back. Flexing your knees whenever you bend or lift provides similar assistance: This flattens the spine and distributes body weight between your back and legs.

Yet no matter how careful you are, there are times—whether you are engaging in vigorous sports or simply hoisting a child into a crib—when you cannot avoid placing extra strain on the lower back. To provide your back with a reserve of strength and flexibility that will allow it to meet such demands without suffering damage, try the exercises shown on pages 64-65.

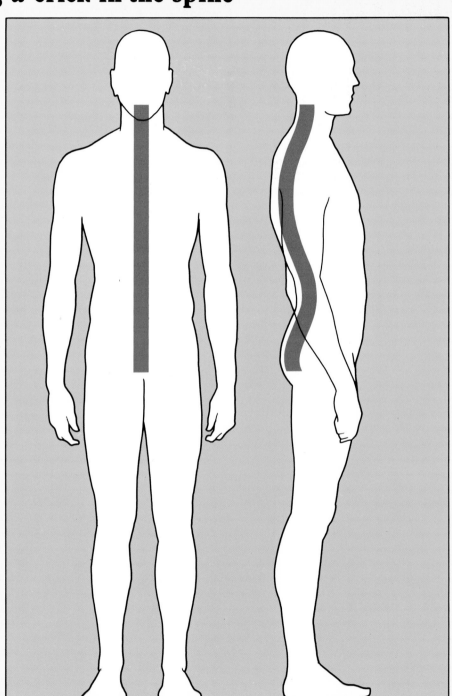

POSTURE FOR A PAIN-FREE BACK
A healthy spine viewed from the front appears as a straight, vertical column; from the side, it forms a relaxed S curve. To maintain this alignment, hold your head up, keep your shoulders even, and balance your pelvis directly over your legs.

HOW TO STAND

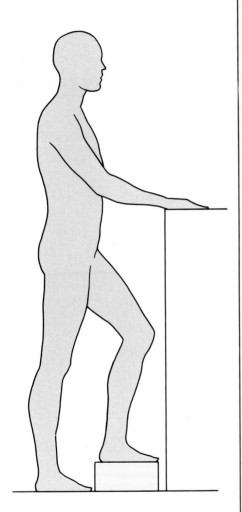

THE VALUE OF RESTING ONE FOOT
When standing for prolonged periods, follow the example of barflies and prop a foot on a low stool or rail. This will flex your hips and help keep your lower back and pelvis from sagging into a painful arch.

HOW TO BEND

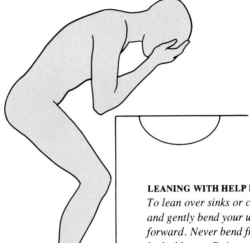

LEANING WITH HELP FROM THE KNEES
To lean over sinks or counters, flex knees and gently bend your upper back forward. Never bend from the waist with locked knees: Doing so places excess strain on your lower back.

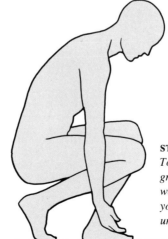

STOOPING SAFELY BY SQUATTING
To bend to the floor, flex your knees and gradually let your legs carry your body weight downward. Tilt your pelvis to round your lower back; you can place one foot under your buttock for balance.

PICKING UP PACKAGES WITHOUT PAIN

Squat down and grasp the object close to your body. Stand up slowly, keeping your pelvis tucked in and using your legs—not your back—to lift the load. Carry it close to your waist—lifting it higher or extending it forward will arch and strain your back. To turn, move your entire body; do not twist your torso.

HANDLING A ONE-ARM LOAD

To carry a suitcase, reach down to the handle by flexing your knees and leaning forward slightly at the waist; keep your back straight. Lift your body upright with your legs and keep your shoulders level, holding your free arm out for balance. To relieve the lopsided pressure, periodically switch sides.

LIFTING AND CARRYING

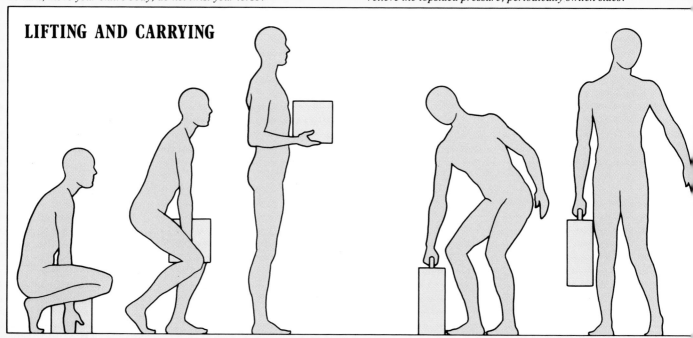

SITTING

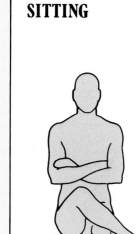
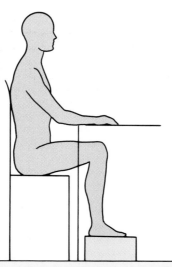
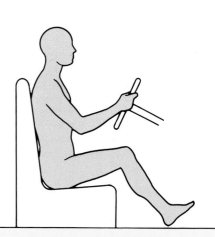

COMFORT FROM CROSSED LEGS

When seated, cross your legs and keep your lower back straight. Recross legs frequently to equalize pressure on hips and legs. Fold your arms to keep their weight from pulling your shoulders forward.

STRATEGIES FOR DESK WORKERS

To ease hours at a desk, rest both feet on a box or stool high enough to raise your knees above your hips, reducing the curve in your lower back. Position your lower spine near the rear of the chair.

A POSTURE FOR SAFE DRIVING

Move the car seat forward so your knees rest higher than your hips. On long drives, make periodic rest stops to stretch your legs and relieve your spine of the subtle but steady pounding of road shock.

BACKPACKING FOR BALANCE
Suspend any object that you will have to carry for an extended time in a harness or a pack that balances the load on your shoulders. This will not overload the lower spine, which is more vulnerable.

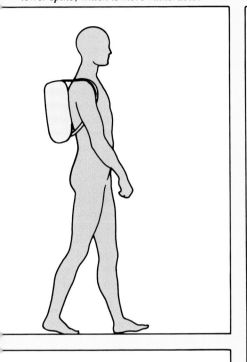

RECLINING

A STRETCH FOR RELAXING
Stretching out on a reclining chair, tipped to elevate your knees above your hips, will soothe an aching back and rest a healthy one. Alternatively, lie flat on the floor with your head on a cushion and your knees bent. Avoid lying on your stomach—especially if you have back pain. If you must do so, place a small pillow beneath your hips to straighten and support your lower spine.

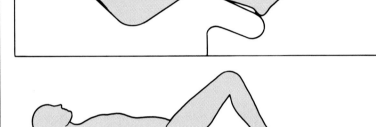

TWO WAYS TO SLEEP
Sleep either on your back with your head on one pillow and your knees crooked over a second one, or on your side with your head on a pillow just large enough to keep your spine straight. If you have a backache, adopt either position, but place a pillow between your thighs as well to keep your pelvis still. Try not to sleep on your stomach: Your spine will sag in the middle.

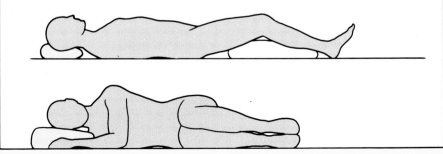

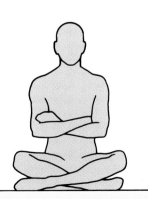

THE BEST SEAT: THE FLOOR
The least stressful way to sit is cross-legged on the floor. Lower yourself gradually, placing one leg in front of the other. Fold your arms. This position subjects your spine to less pressure than sitting in a chair.

Exercising aches away—for good

The exercises on these two pages are among those most commonly recommended by doctors as insurance against backache. They fall into two distinct groups. The three on this page and the first on the facing page are frequently prescribed to rehabilitate an ailing back; they gently stretch and tone the muscles that support the spine. The three that follow are designed to strengthen an already healthy back. Caution: If you have back pain at present or if you have had it in the past, do not attempt the three strengthening exercises, and check with your doctor before trying the others.

At first, do each exercise only three or four times. Because each movement serves as a warm-up for the one that follows, do them in sequence, starting with the preliminary stretch at top left and proceeding to the difficult leg lift at bottom right. Move slowly and deliberately, breathing rhythmically throughout. Stop immediately if you feel any pain: You could be injuring yourself. Some stiffness or awkwardness at first is normal and need cause no alarm. Simply extend each movement only so far as comfortable. As you become stronger and more flexible, your stamina and range of motion will increase. Eventually, you should work up to 25 repetitions of each exercise in a daily 8- to 10-minute routine.

ROLLING OUT THE KINKS

To begin a back exercise routine, sit on a hard chair, feet flat on the floor and arms dangling. Roll forward from the waist, your hands toward your ankles, your head between your knees. Go only so far as comfortable, then hold that position for six seconds and slowly roll upright.

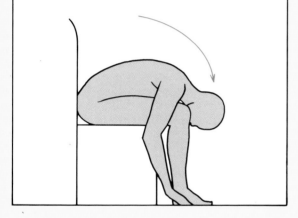

TILTING THE PELVIS FOR A STRAIGHT, FLEXIBLE SPINE

Lie on your back with your knees bent, your hands folded behind your head. Inhale, then breathe out, at the same time tightening your buttocks and contracting stomach muscles to press your lower back (straight arrow) against the floor; your pelvis will tilt upward (curved arrow) slightly. Hold for six seconds, breathing normally, then relax and repeat.

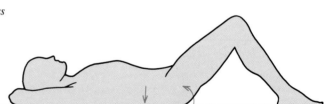

MODIFIED SIT-UPS FOR A STRONG STOMACH

Lie on your back, palms at your side, pelvis tilted upward slightly. With your arms outstretched, lift your head and shoulders and reach for your knees. Hold for six seconds, then roll down, pressing the small of your back against the floor. Once you can perform this exercise with ease, begin bringing your entire torso up, first with your arms folded across your chest, eventually with your hands clasped behind your head.

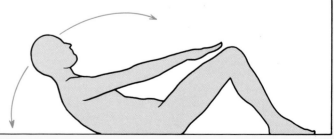

STRETCHING THE MUSCLES ALONG THE SPINE
Lying in the position sketched in the center drawing at left, clasp both hands around one knee and pull it toward your chest, simultaneously curling your head and shoulders forward. Hold for six seconds, then unroll to the original position; repeat with the opposite leg. After this exercise becomes easy, pull both legs to your chest at the same time.

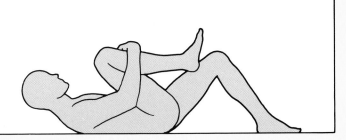

A MODIFIED PUSH-UP TO STRENGTHEN A HEALTHY BACK
Lie on your stomach with your elbows bent, palms flat on the floor next to your shoulders. Using your arms, push your upper body up as far as you can comfortably, then lower yourself to the floor. Keep your thighs, knees and toes pressed to the floor. Caution: Do not continue this exercise if it causes pain.

ALTERNATE LEG RAISES
Lying on your stomach, arms to the side, raise one leg completely off the floor—keeping it straight if possible, bending your knee if not. Hold for a few seconds, then lower your leg and repeat the exercise with the opposite one. When you have completed this exercise, roll immediately onto your back and pull your knees to your chest to stretch your lower spine.

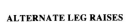

LEG LIFTS THAT STRENGTHEN THE STOMACH
Lie on your back, hands either beneath your buttocks to help support your lower back, or at your sides. Simultaneously raise both legs six inches off the floor; hold that position for up to five seconds, then return your legs to the floor. After completing the exercise, pull your knees to your chest. Caution: This is a strenuous exercise that can severely strain a weak back; do not attempt it if you have even minor backache.

Best foot forward

Although his head was generally preoccupied with speculation on logic and morality, the Greek philosopher Socrates kept his feet on the ground. A practical man of modest tastes, he habitually spent his days walking Athens' streets barefoot. On several occasions when he served with the Athenian army, his capacity for marching unshod over icy terrain dumfounded those about him; he bore up better than most soldiers who were wearing shoes. Still, this wise man was no stranger to the ills of the foot. "To him whose feet hurt," he was reputed to have remarked, "everything hurts."

In truth, the feet—the stepchildren of the human body and the butt of jokes since time immemorial—can critically affect a person's well-being. The most inconsequential foot maladies not only can mirror or cause larger problems elsewhere in the body but can by themselves swiftly alter a mood.

Intricate mechanisms, the feet are designed not only to balance and support the body but to propel it at many speeds on all sorts of surfaces. The typical worker walks up to seven and a half miles a day, a busy housekeeper close to 10 miles, subjecting the foot to a cumulative impact estimated at several hundred tons. The average person walks some 70,000 miles in a lifetime, almost three trips around the globe.

For most of those miles his feet give him no reason to notice them. Yet at one time or another, huge numbers of people become painfully aware of their feet. About 50 per cent of all adults say their feet hurt. The causes are basic. One derives from humans' method of walking on two legs instead of four: The prehuman hind feet once supported only half the body weight; now human legs carry it all. The impact is increased when feet pound against concrete instead of a grassy meadow. A second cause is of greater import. The graceful and generally faultless feet are forced out of shape by ill-fitting shoes, which keep them from supporting their load naturally. This distortion twists bones and nails, strains muscles and ligaments, and abrades the skin so it forms projecting calluses, or corns. Also, shoes block air circulation, promoting attacks by fungi. In a typical year in the United States alone, the footsore made 35 million visits to medical practitioners and spent $136 million on medication.

What humankind has done to its feet, however, it can undo. Returning to a four-legged stance or bare feet is impractical, but the commonest foot ailments can be averted by good hygiene, correct posture and gait, and well-fitting shoes. Serious disorders can often be banished by exercises or corrective footwear. Minor annoyances, such as fungus infection, can be eliminated with effective new medicines.

The feet require care because they are complicated structures. They contain more than a quarter of all the bones in the body—26 each. The key bone is the cubical anklebone, or talus, which is gripped securely between the knobby lower ends of the two leg bones to form the ankle joint. The talus moves up and down on an axis between those knobs. One of the many surprising facts about the foot is that, although the ankle knobs of each foot may seem identically placed, the inside one is above and considerably forward of its companion on the outer side. The axis tilts. When the foot moves

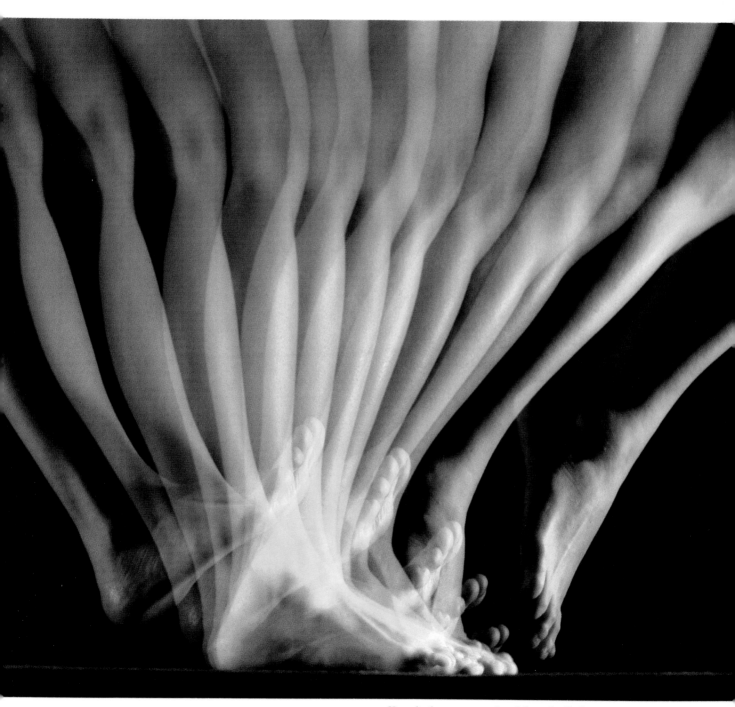

How the foot manages the tricky task of balancing and propelling
the body is traced in this multiple exposure of a single step. The
heel takes the body's weight first; then the foot swings down and
the load shifts to the base of the little toe, then to the ball of the
foot, and finally off the foot with the spring of the big toe.

upward on this oblique hinge it naturally toes out slightly to the side; and when the foot is extended to take a forward step it generally inclines outward; thus the outer edge of the heel is the point that first strikes the ground.

To this obliquely rotating anklebone are attached strong projections to both rear and front. Out and down to the rear juts the heel, or calcaneus, bone, the foot's largest. Although it absorbs the most merciless pounding, it can do so and adjust to odd surfaces because it is connected to the anklebone by a joint that enables it to move slightly from side to side. To observe this flexibility, grab your ankle firmly with one hand and note the extent to which you can waggle your heel sideways with the other.

Projecting forward from the front of the heel are a group of seven irregularly shaped bones known collectively as the tarsus, the Greek word for wicker basket, which their intricate arrangement somewhat resembles. Each is connected to its neighbor by a joint allowing slight movement and providing the foot with its amazing elasticity. The tarsal bones and the talus function more or less as does the wrist, making possible sideways as well as up-and-down motions. The tarsal bones also form the top of the arch, supported in the rear by the heel bone and in the front by five metatarsal bones, one for each toe. These descend from the tarsus to form the ball of the foot. Most of them can flex up or down, the first and fifth more than the others. Out beyond the metatarsals extend the toe bones—two in the big toe and three in the others (paralleling the structure of the fingers).

In addition there are tiny sesamoid bones—so called because they resemble sesame seeds—but they are not usually counted in the tally of human bones because their number may vary from two to four. Imbedded in the foot underneath the base of the big toe, the sesamoids help form an arch that keeps that part of the toe off the ground, creating a tunnel for tendons to pass through without being pinched. These tendons in turn enable the big toe to flex upward easily—as it does about 900 times with every mile walked.

Holding the foot's structure together is a host of ligaments, about 125, and powering it is a network of some 38 muscles. One conglomeration of ligaments plays a particularly impor-

tant role. That is the plantar fascia, a tough band with the consistency of a rubber tire, two to three inches wide and more than a quarter of an inch thick; it forms the biggest part of the sole of the foot, protecting the softer muscles of the foot and helping to hold the arch in proper tension.

How to walk smoothly

Each step, as a matter of fact, summons into coordinated action virtually every bone and muscle in the foot—as well as many others above it. Two aspects of the motion—pronating and supinating—are responsible for much of the smoothness and adaptability of the human walk. Pronating means turning downward and inward; supinating means turning upward and outward. In the course of a single stride the foot shifts automatically from pronating to supinating and back again. This series of motions begins when a normal foot hits the ground on the outside of the heel. The foot then pronates, rolling down and inward, and the arch lowers a little. Flexing toward the ground, the foot rotates the toes toward the inside so that they face more or less straight ahead. All this is necessary so that the foot, helped by motion of the ankle, can adapt swiftly to the surface it is striking.

A split second later the scene changes drastically as the foot abandons its role of sensitive ground-feeler and becomes a powerful launching device. After landing firmly and bearing the full weight of the body, the foot begins the series of upward and outward movements called supination. First the heel comes off the ground, and the foot becomes rigid in order to provide the stability needed to lift the body and propel it. Then the arch rises. The last part of the foot to leave the ground will be the big toe—the body's full weight having been transferred, during the stride, from the outside of the heel to the strongest toe.

As the foot moves up and down through supinating and pronating, the knee hinge swings back and forth while the pelvis moves in three directions at once: It swivels, like a turntable, to follow the limbs as they swing to and fro; it tilts up and down, like a seesaw; and it shuttles from side to side as the body's weight is shifted first over one leg and then the other. The combined movements of all these parts of the

What makes feet hurt

The human foot can support high loads and stresses—the weight of the body and the shocks of walking and jumping—over a lifetime because of its uniquely strong, resilient structure. Its arch is really a series of arches, curving in two directions, from ball to heel and from side to side, and giving the foot great load-bearing capacity; and the arch is articulated, made up of many small bones that can shift relative to one another to absorb the blows of movement. So long as this healthy structure *(below)* is maintained, the footaches of sightseeing or hiking disappear with rest. But chronic stress—caused by the extra weight of obesity or by continuous standing on the job—can eventually alter the healthy structure *(below, right)*, so distorting it that the feet hurt chronically.

The aching and burning of chronic foot strain arise because excess stress and weight stretch the ligaments connecting the bones, inflaming them so that they hurt. If the strain continues, the ligaments deteriorate, losing their ability to pull the bones back into the proper positions. The most common result is a permanent inward tilting of the ankle. Temporary tilting is necessary in walking, but ordinarily the ankle springs back up; when it does not, the foot flattens out, losing the strength and resilience of the arch.

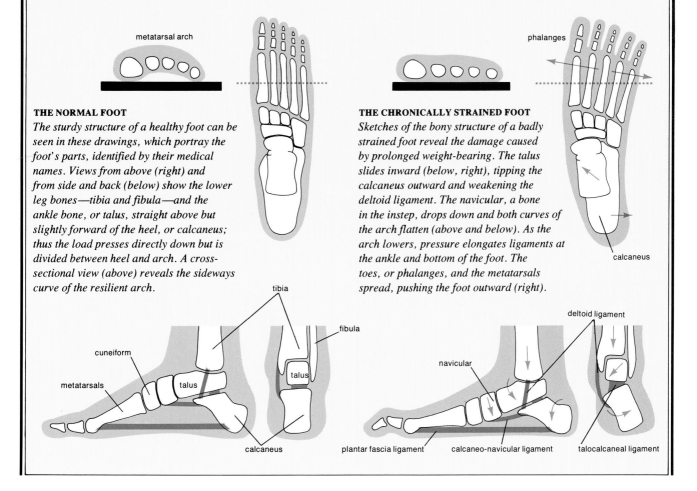

metatarsal arch

phalanges

THE NORMAL FOOT
The sturdy structure of a healthy foot can be seen in these drawings, which portray the foot's parts, identified by their medical names. Views from above (right) and from side and back (below) show the lower leg bones—tibia and fibula—and the ankle bone, or talus, straight above but slightly forward of the heel, or calcaneus; thus the load presses directly down but is divided between heel and arch. A cross-sectional view (above) reveals the sideways curve of the resilient arch.

THE CHRONICALLY STRAINED FOOT
Sketches of the bony structure of a badly strained foot reveal the damage caused by prolonged weight-bearing. The talus slides inward (below, right), tipping the calcaneus outward and weakening the deltoid ligament. The navicular, a bone in the instep, drops down and both curves of the arch flatten (above and below). As the arch lowers, pressure elongates ligaments at the ankle and bottom of the foot. The toes, or phalanges, and the metatarsals spread, pushing the foot outward (right).

calcaneus

tibia

fibula

cuneiform

talus

talus

metatarsals

deltoid ligament

navicular

calcaneus

plantar fascia ligament

calcaneo-navicular ligament

talocalcaneal ligament

frame create a gait unique to each person. But some gaits are more memorable than others: the waddle of Charlie Chaplin's tramp, for instance, the mesmerizing movement of Marilyn Monroe, or the rolling amble of John Wayne.

Gaits vary from one culture to another because they are learned by children, who mimic their parents. Babies born blind, found Eileen P. Scott of the Canadian National Institute of the Blind, never try to stand and walk spontaneously; they have to be taught. Many Japanese women walk with a mincing gait, and women of India sway their hips more than most Western women. ''American women,'' observed one disapproving Indian male, ''walk like men.''

Walking is also influenced by footwear. In France three brother orthopedists, Drs. Robert, Jean and Pierre Ducroquet, watched and photographed people from all walks of life as they paced up and down a runway. Among the doctors' findings: Women—who already walk with a slightly sway-backed posture to balance the weight of their breasts—accentuate the lower-back curvature and take shorter steps when they put on high-heeled shoes. The Ducroquets also filmed the clumping gait of a sewer worker wearing his work clothes and heavy leather boots. ''The folds of his boots show clearly that the man must struggle against the rigidity of his enormous constriction,'' they noted, ''not only at the level of his foot, but also at the level of his knees.'' With his normal forward thrust hampered by the big boots, the man had to throw his legs out to the side to lurch ahead.

Some styles of walking may be not only more graceful but also more beneficial than others. Comfortable shoes, upright posture and rhythmic motion make walking more efficient. When the head is held high and the trunk upright, the chest can expand fully with each breath, so walking is not fatiguing. The arms should swing naturally at the sides, opposite to the motion of the legs. The legs should first propel, then pull the body through each step; they should not let the whole frame fall lazily forward, plunking the body's weight down on each foot. Whether the feet are pointed straight forward or toe in or out a little does not seem to matter. Keeping the feet parallel has long been advocated by many doctors as the ideal, but when Dr. Dudley J. Morton of Columbia University conducted tests on Africans who were free of foot ailments, he found that the majority of them walked with their toes directed outward.

Exercises that benefit the feet

Keeping the feet strong, flexible and ready to withstand a hard day's pounding is fairly simple. It requires attention to the routines of daily hygiene, some special exercises, and shoes and stockings chosen for fit and the practical characteristics of their materials.

The feet get the best exercise simply from a brisk walk in well-fitting footwear. But some extra exercises can help strengthen muscles and keep the feet from getting weary. Begin by first shaking or massaging the feet (opposite) to loosen tight muscles. Then move on to these routines:
● Sitting on the floor, point the feet straight ahead, curl the toes under and, keeping the heels on the floor, turn the feet to point toward each other. Hold this position for a count of two, then relax and repeat the movement 10 times.
● Lying either in bed or on the floor, bend the toes first down, then up 10 times.
● Drop a handful of marbles on the floor and pick them up with the toes. What might seem child's play is an effective muscle-building exercise.
● To strengthen the supporting tendons and ligaments of the ankle, lie on your back, extend the right leg and make a circle

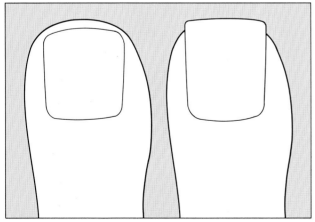

Surprisingly important to foot care is trimming the toenails; they should be cut as shown at right above: straight across and long enough so the nail covers the skin. Incorrect trimming —short and curving (left)—can make the nail grow into tender skin or push skin aside, causing a painful ingrown nail.

with the foot in a counterclockwise direction. Repeat the circular motion with the left foot but in a clockwise direction. Perform the exercise 10 times for each foot, being sure all the motion is in the ankle, not the knee or the hip.

The hygiene of foot care is not as simple as it might seem. Trim toenails straight across and not close to the skin *(opposite)*. Cutting toenails around the edges and too close to the quick—the growing portion of the nail bed—may cause a corner of the nail to become embedded in the flesh and, if the toe is jammed between the side of a tight shoe and another toe, this skin flap can become inflamed and even infected. Caught early, such an ingrown toenail that is not infected can be treated effectively at home by soaking the foot in warm water, then working wisps of absorbent cotton under the nail corner with a manicure orange stick.

Equally important is washing feet daily with soap and water, drying them well and keeping them dry. Dryness curbs not only infections but the embarrassing condition called bromidrosis, a polite way of saying smelly feet.

Though shoes influence many foot ills, other ailments are caused by infection or by slight structural abnormalities. The commonest infections, one from a virus and one from fungi, are hard to avoid but fairly readily treated. The plantar wart, which looks like a callus on the bottom of the foot, is actually a benign tumor caused by the papilloma virus. An adult's plantar wart can be left alone if it does not hurt; it may

disappear spontaneously in a few weeks. If it is painful, treat it like a corn, soaking the foot in warm water and rubbing the wart with a pumice stone. In children, these warts spread rapidly, so they should be treated right away by a doctor.

Less painful but annoying is that scourge of locker rooms and swimming pools around the world, athlete's foot, an infection from any of several species of fungus commonly called ringworm. Sores form between the toes and frequently on the bottom of the feet, and the skin peels and itches. Most victims are men—according to one source, some eight out of 10 men are troubled by athlete's foot. The infection can often be forestalled by keeping the toes clean and dry.

Preventing trouble from fungus

Prevention of athlete's foot is important because the fungus is a constant companion of human life. It is always present on everyone's skin, but it may cause infection only once in a while—or never. The infections can be eliminated from most spots by applying any of a number of nonprescription fungicides. Those with labels specifying that they contain either undecylenic acid or tolnaftate have been deemed safe and effective by government advisory panels. However, these topical fungicides can harm the skin if applied under nails and in hairy areas—where infections may persist. Even such resistant cases can be cured by an antifungus pill, griseofulvin, but it may have to be taken regularly for months

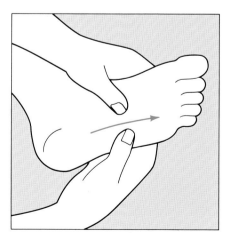

The easy-to-learn foot massage portrayed in these three drawings can relieve muscle tension. To begin, grasp the sole between thumbs and fingers (above). Starting at the heel, press against the sole with thumbs, moving forward gradually toward the toes.

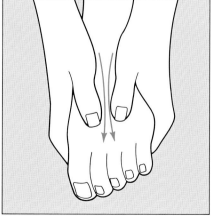

To massage the top of the foot, hold the foot with both hands—thumbs on top, fingertips on the sole. Starting high on the instep, near the shin, exert firm, pulsing pressure with thumbs and the heels of the hands. Work forward from the ankle to the toes.

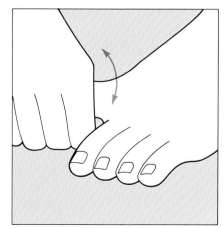

To complete the foot massage, wrap fingers around the big toe and gently pull on it. Slowly twist the hand (not the toe) back and forth, sliding it out gradually toward the tip of the toe. Repeat for each toe. Then massage the other foot.

and it sometimes causes allergic reactions or stomach upsets.

Controlling moisture to prevent infection is no small task because the average adult's feet have, by one estimate, 250,000 sweat glands that pour out moisture at the rate of about a half pint a day, and some people's feet sweat even more than that. Powdering the feet with talcum powder or foot powder is helpful.

Feet will also stay drier if they are clad in socks and shoes that allow them to breathe. The most effective hosiery is the kind that will draw perspiration away from the feet as a wick does kerosene from the base of a lamp. Natural fibers—cotton and silk—meet this requirement better than synthetic materials do, according to foot specialists with the Pennsylvania College of Podiatric Medicine. The excellent absorbency of these natural fibers seems to present problems only for runners, who complain that their sweat-soaked socks become too heavy and slow them down.

Shoes, too, are a key to keeping feet dry, for their material and construction determine how readily they allow moisture and heat to escape from the feet. They are essential to all foot care, but they are also at the bottom of much foot trouble, making them a necessary evil of the urban life that comes with civilization.

Historically, shoes were first required to protect the feet in cities and towns, where grassy paths were replaced by heavily traveled walkways; the traffic—then simply foot traffic—pounded the ground into a hard, unyielding surface. If the route was paved to eliminate mud, it became harder yet. Such walkways—made rough by an occasional pebble—painfully battered bare feet. By about 2000 B.C., Egyptians were cushioning their feet with flat sandals of woven reeds or leather. In northern Europe, this open sandal evolved into an enclosing shoe to shield the foot from cold—the extremities, which expose more surface area per unit of volume than other parts of the body, lose vital heat quickly and freeze easily.

But from the beginning, practical considerations for foot protection have often given way to a passion for foot decoration that persists today. There is a tale, perhaps apocryphal, of a woman who dreamed she was strolling down the street as naked as the emperor without his clothes—except that she was wearing shoes. When she related this troubling vision to her psychiatrist, he probed, ''And you felt embarrassed?'' ''Terribly,'' she confessed. ''They were last year's shoes.''

The concern for fashion is ancient. In Rome, tradition dictated who should wear what color: Julius Caesar was once criticized for wearing red boots considered more fitting for a younger man. By the 11th and 12th Centuries, European dandies put on slippers with toes turned up and twisted to resemble rams' horns, and by the 15th Century, upturned toes reached such absurd lengths that courtiers had to hold them up with silk straps and gold chains in order to avoid tripping over them. In that same era European aristocrats also elevated themselves on platform shoes called *chopines,* which reached heights of 30 inches. To remain upright, women required long staffs or the supporting arms of their maids. Because pregnant women often suffered miscarriages when they toppled off their *chopines,* Venice passed a law in 1430 prohibiting them from wearing the dangerous fashion—to little avail.

The modern versions of *chopines* cause similar hazards. When the platform style reappeared in the early 1970s doctors reported an increase in foot injuries and broken legs. Dr. Seymour Frank of the New York College of Podiatric Medicine said he saw six to eight foot injuries each week directly attributable to platform shoes. ''Once the sole becomes so thick that the foot loses contact with the ground, you've got a problem,'' he explained. ''A lot of information the brain receives concerning the sense of orientation with the ground comes from nerves in the sole of the foot; without them you can throw off your sense of balance.''

If platform soles put the feet out of touch with the ground, a woman's stylish party shoes, with soles only ⅛ inch thick, fail to cushion the feet at all. A far better compromise is the sole of a businessman's shoe, ¼ inch thick, although someone who must consistently pound the pavement would be better served by a thicker sole—a letter carrier's shoe is made with soles an inch thick.

Platform soles, like other extremes of shoe fashion, are popular only briefly and intermittently, but other design characteristics equally bad for the feet persist. Shoes are made too narrow, too short and too sharply angled to properly house the normal human foot. And often, the material selected is not the most appropriate.

Choosing comfortable shoes

Shoe bottoms can be made of any material that is flexible and cushiony but firm. Leather, plastics and rubber serve well. Rigid materials, such as the wood often used for clogs, interfere with a normal gait and may cause irritating friction. For shoe ''uppers''—everything above the sole—leather is still the first choice because it breathes; its natural pores permit moisture and heat to escape and help keep the feet dry. Plain canvas uppers—commonly used for tennis and running shoes and frequently worn by children—also breathe well; running shoes made of a cotton-nylon blend are slightly less porous. Most synthetics, even those specially made to be porous, cannot yet equal leather or canvas in breathability.

Leather offers the added advantage of holding its shape. It is firm enough to give support to bones and muscles but pliable enough to flex with the foot; eventually it gives, conforming to the shape of the individual foot and achieving the comfort of an old shoe. No other material can do as well.

New shoes are often uncomfortable, but they need not be. The most comfortable are those shaped to copy the contours of the foot—as are army boots, which were designed to ease walking, protect the feet and prevent blisters and other painful ailments. In the 1950s the U.S. Army surveyed 10,000 soldiers, measuring their feet and asking about their foot comfort. The study noted the different physical details of their feet as well as how heavy a load they usually carried and how much their feet swelled during the day.

The data were used to design the boot that became standard issue. It is wide at the toe so the bones there do not squeeze together, and narrow at the heel to prevent slippage during movement. And of course the heel is low—just ⅞ inch. A lower heel may shift weight, straining the body's entire bone structure. A higher heel makes balance precarious and slides the foot forward in the shoe, loosening its grip on the heel so that the foot slips and rubs there while the toes squeeze against the front of the shoe. Laced calf-high, the

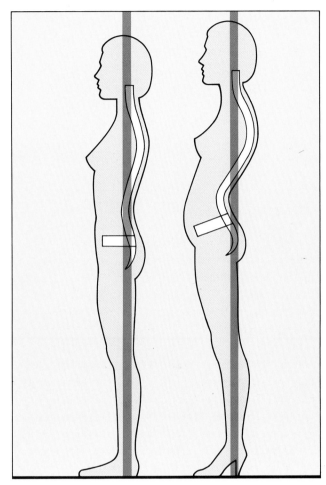

Why high-heeled shoes make the back and legs hurt is indicated in these drawings. High heels tip the body forward (right), accentuating the natural curve of the spine indicated in the left sketch. The tipping forces the wearer to maintain balance by thrusting the shoulders back from the center line (vertical bar), causing the abdomen to protrude, the pelvis to tilt forward and the knees to flex imperceptibly. In addition, the calf muscles eventually shorten and weaken.

army boot holds the foot snugly to protect the ankle, and a heavy sole provides excellent shock absorption and grip.

The shape of any shoe is determined by a form known as a last, over which individual pieces of leather are stitched. The last is not a replica of a foot but rather a simulation of what people want the foot to look like. As fashions fluctuate, the shapes of the lasts used to manufacture shoes also change, toes being broadened, rounded, tapered or pointed, heels elevated or lowered. Originally lasts were hand-carved of wood—hard maple was a favorite. Today machines, computer-programed with the measurements for manufacturers' myriad lasts, turn out lasts of plastic, preferred over wood because it will not shrink or swell with temperature or humidity changes during the shoemaking process.

Because the last establishes the final shape of a shoe, it also sets the size. In the United States, Britain and some other countries, shoe sizes are calibrated in thirds of an inch—about the length of one dried barleycorn. This unusual unit of measure was chosen by King Edward I, who in 1305 decreed that three barleycorns would measure an inch and that a child's shoe that measured 13 barleycorns would be size 13. King Edward's system also applies to adult shoes—a man's size 10 is $1/3$ inch longer than a size 9. Most European countries, however, use a system based on metrics. In France, Italy, Spain and elsewhere shoes are scaled by $2/3$ centimeter; thus a size 40 shoe is $2/3$ centimeter—$1/4$ inch—longer than a size 39. In most countries width is indicated by letter systems. In the United States a size 8B is $1/4$ inch wider than an 8A across the ball of the foot and proportionately larger in every dimension except length.

Each size in each style requires its own last. At one time American manufacturers used some 300 lasts, in lengths from an infant's 0 to a man's 16 and widths from the very narrow AAAAA to EEEEE. There were many "combination lasts" having one width for the heel and another for the toe.

Rules for a good fit

That wide range of sizes has become increasingly uncommon, and inexpensive shoes may be available only in a single average width called medium. Still, so many kinds of shoes are made on a great variety of lasts that almost anyone can find shoes that fit comfortably by following a few common-sense rules:

● Shop for shoes late in the day rather than early, because feet swell as the day passes and shoes must accommodate the enlargement; wear hosiery suited to the shoes—it is pointless to try on hiking boots over sheer nylons.

● Because almost everyone has one foot larger than the other, try on both shoes of a pair and settle on the size fitting the larger foot—extra roominess is better than tightness.

● Standing up with weight on the foot, check the space in the "toe box" in front by wiggling the toes and pressing down on the box with a finger; there should be at least half an inch of free space ahead of the longest toe.

● Check the location of the ball of the foot; it should be in the widest part of the shoe to avoid cramping the toes.

● Walk around on an uncarpeted floor to make sure the back of the shoe grips the heelbone firmly without squeezing; slight slippage—which will probably disappear as wear makes the sole flexible—is acceptable.

● Because lasts vary so much, try on several sizes, not just the size ordinarily worn; it may even be necessary to try on several different pairs of the same size—the way leather pieces are assembled introduces subtle alterations in shape that affect comfort.

● When a pair of shoes turns out to be exceptionally comfortable, remember the name of the manufacturer; the lasts are unusually well suited to your foot and such shoes are worth looking for.

Although well-fitting shoes help everyone, they are of special importance to certain people: to the elderly, whose bones and muscles weaken with age; to diabetics, who risk great danger from such a simple injury as a blister; and to children, whose feet are growing and malleable. The bones of very young children are so soft they will conform to the shape of an ill-chosen shoe, rather than the other way around. And they grow so rapidly that to make sure shoes are not overtight, frequent, regular measurement is necessary: every two months up to the age of six, every three months to the age of 10 and every four months to the age of 12.

The painful price of a poor fit

The comic-strip author who wrote ''If the shoe fits, podiatrists are out of work'' was not far off the mark. Many of the 28 million visits Americans pay to foot doctors each year are occasioned by the wearing of shoes that, instead of conforming to the contours of the foot, skimp on room at some trouble spots and leave too much of it at others. Some common shoe-fitting errors are illustrated here: toe boxes too narrow or short, inadequate fit along the arch, and heels too tight or too loose.

The key to avoiding such trouble is the position of the ball of the foot, the pivotal weight-bearing point indicated in the drawings by the large blue circles. Because it is at the broadest point of the foot, the ball should always fit into the widest part of the shoe. But it often falls farther forward, pushed there by a shoe that is too short *(below)* or too long *(right)*, or by a high heel. This improper position may also leave the arch unsupported and lead to foot strain. The fact that women suffer four times as many foot problems as men is attributed largely to the deleterious effects of high heels, which throw a disproportionate amount of weight forward.

THE PINCH OF POINTED SHOES
The ball of the foot in the sketch below rests forward of its natural position—the shoe's widest point—crowding the rest of the foot. Toes that overlap this way may develop corns, ingrown toenails and the joint deformations called bunions.

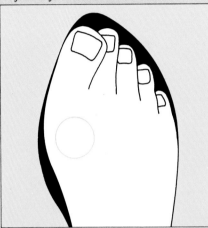

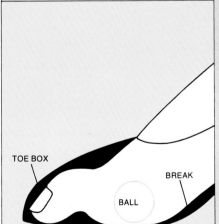

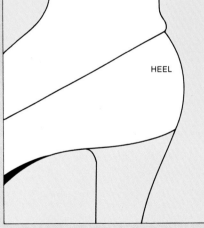

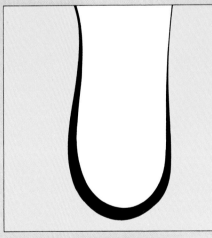

TOES JAMMED IN A SHORT TOE BOX
Because the ball of the foot pictured here does not settle firmly into the so-called break of the shoe, the foot can slide forward, jamming toes so they rub against the shoe's inner surface. Hammertoes, corns and calluses may result.

SQUEEZE FROM A HEEL
A heel that, like this one, grips too tightly squeezes the tendon out above the heel. The two-inch heel pictured is the maximum height advised. Higher ones invite woes, from calluses on the soles to back pain caused by a strained gait.

THE WOBBLE OF A LOOSE HEEL
The most obvious effect of a heel as loose as this one is blisters caused by up-and-down friction. Heels leaving a gap between foot and shoe can also cause side-to-side instability, throwing the weight forward and creating a wobbling gait.

called corns. "And when too short the modish shoes are worn," rhymed the 18th Century English poet John Gay, "You'll judge the seasons by your shooting corn." Representing the body's attempt to protect itself against the frictions and pressures of cramping shoes or of socks that bunch up at the toe or the heel, corns are small build-ups of dead skin—white or yellow, either waxy or dry and hard, with a deep central core. They generally develop on the tops of toes, although soft corns may also appear between toes. Somewhat similar but larger calluses are found on the ball of the foot or around the heel. Calluses are the second most prevalent chronic condition—after arthritis—of the body's bones and joints.

Theodorice, the Bishop of Cervia in northern Italy, described one remedy in 1267: "Callused flesh should be excavated all around, and then extirpated down to its roots with forceps or scissors or some other instrument. Afterward, the spot should be cauterized and cared for until it heals." The bishop's basic method is used today and probably causes more foot pain than it heals—the danger of infection is great, and a wrong move can produce serious bleeding.

There are safer ways to remove corns. Drugstores sell "corn plasters" and similar medicines that contain mild acids to dissolve dead skin; they have been found by a government review panel to be safe if applications are limited to five treatments over two weeks. Most foot specialists, however, recommend a milder method: At bedtime soak the foot to soften the dead skin, then rub gently with a pumice stone, available at drugstores. Until a corn or callus disappears, the pain it causes can be relieved with a doughnut-shaped pad, also available at the drugstore.

Bunions, hammertoe and fallen arches

Not so easily cured are ailments that, like corns, are affected by shoes, but arise from minor structural abnormalities: a bunion, a projection that develops at a joint of the big toe; hammertoe, a crook in one of the toe joints; and flat feet, weakness of the arches. All are sometimes painful, and they may detract from appearance.

over the years their ligaments become looser and less supportive, the metatarsal joints separate from one another and the first and biggest is pushed away from its neighbor toward the inside of the foot. Constricting, pointed shoes push the big toe back sharply toward the others. As the jutting metatarsal joint rubs against the inside of the shoe it becomes inflamed and swollen.

If the exposed joint does not push out too far, the problem can be handled simply by wearing wide, comfortable shoes with ample toe space. Sometimes, however, the big-toe joint swells up so much that, even in roomy shoes, the toe pushes toward the middle of the foot and rubs against the neighboring toe, threatening to twist it. In such cases surgery may be needed. Drugstore bunion shields offer scant relief, and improperly worn they might make the bunion worse. But protective padding will relieve pain from a small relative of the bunion—the bunionette—that appears on the opposite side of the foot, on the little toe. It is sometimes called a tailor's bunion because it used to crop up frequently among garment-makers who sat cross-legged on the floor to sew and thus placed pressure on the smallest toe joint.

A quite different deformation of toe joints causes hammertoes—one or more toes curl up or are jammed up until they resemble the hammer that strikes a piano string. The second toe—next to the big toe—is most frequently affected, but its abnormal bending can induce hammering in its neighbors.

Although hammertoes can be inherited—the tendon that pulls on the toe pulls too strongly—they, like corns and bunions, are made worse by ill-fitting shoes, and by hosiery that is too tight. Not surprisingly, hammertoes pain women much more than men because women are more likely to wear shoe styles with pointed toes. The only treatment short of surgery—a routine procedure—is roomy shoes.

Of the foot troubles people are born with, the most common affect the complex interlocking assemblage of bones, muscles and ligaments making up the arch. If the arch is either unusually high or low, it loses some of its capacity to support the weight of the body and absorb the shocks of walking. Such feet tire quickly, and they often hurt. Either of

The science of putting feet back into line

Like car wheels that are out of line, misaligned foot bones—whether the result of a congenital defect or simple wear and tear—can damage themselves and the body they carry. To correct such misalignments, many foot specialists prescribe orthotics, custom-made shoe inserts that maintain the feet at precise heights and angles, realigning the bones and redistributing weight. Because no two feet are precisely alike, making the corrective devices is an exacting process.

Doctors first must scrutinize the patient's gait, sometimes employing treadmills and videotape cameras to get a better look *(below)*. Next, they make impressions of the feet in plaster. The casts, which may be accompanied by instructions based on the doctor's visual diagnosis, are then sent to a specialist, who uses the cast as a mold to fashion the inserts.

The final products vary greatly, not only in height, length and shape but also in composition, hardness and flexibility. A stiff orthotic, for example, might stop an inward turning of the foot that places stress on a knee, while a more flexible insert might be used for someone who can tolerate only a limited amount of correction—such as an elderly person.

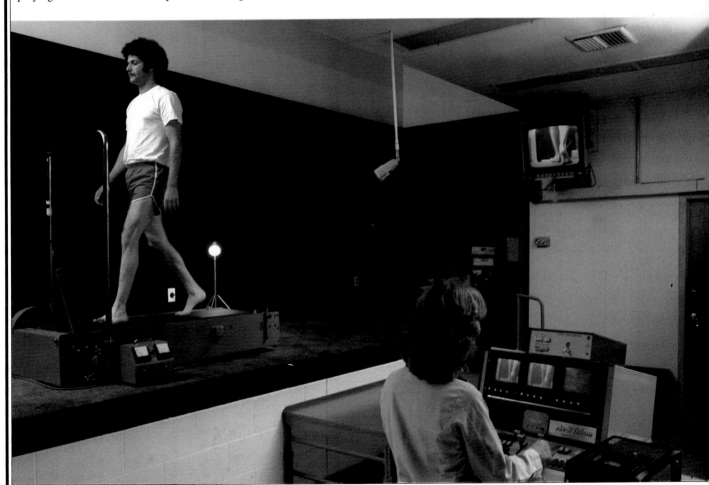

Walking on a treadmill, a patient has his stride videotaped. The large screen at upper right reveals a problem that shoe inserts can correct: The patient's left foot points outward excessively while his right foot tilts inward as the heel rises.

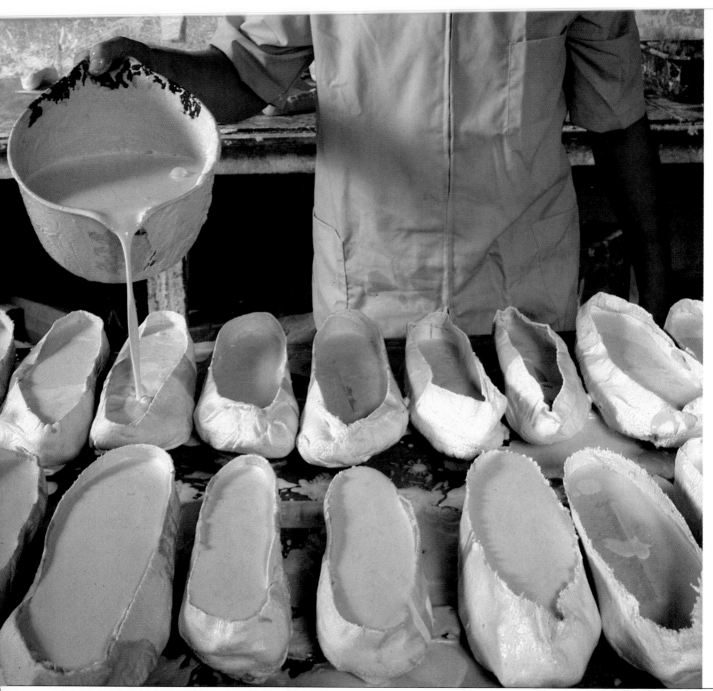

Liquid plaster is poured into a mold of a patient's foot, making a replica of the lower portion. Onto that replica is pressed a hot sheet of plastic that forms an orthotic shell—an impression of the foot to be built up as specified by the doctor for the patient's use.

A technician spreads gummy plastic on the heel of the shell (red) for a patient's left foot. Before it hardens, it is shaped. At left, a measuring device reveals that an orthotic under a mold of a patient's right foot will angle it as required—four degrees.

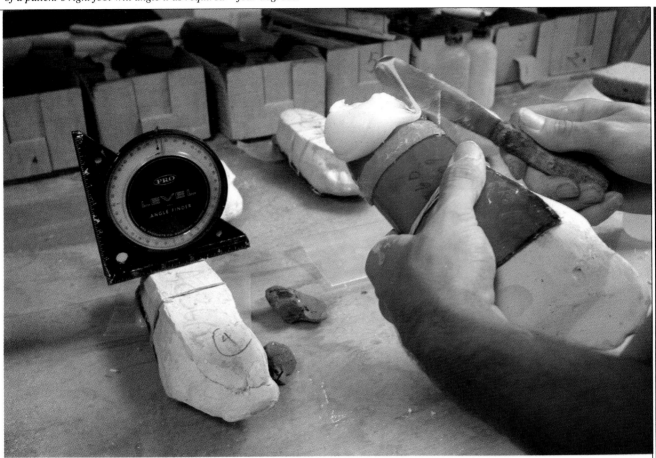

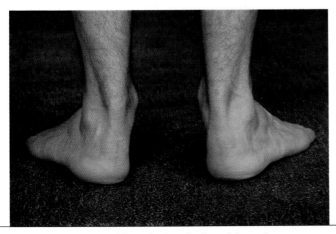

Before being corrected by orthotics, the feet of the patient on the treadmill (page 77) show the effects of bone misalignment: They tilt inward severely, causing his body's weight to fall on the inner edge rather than the center of each heel.

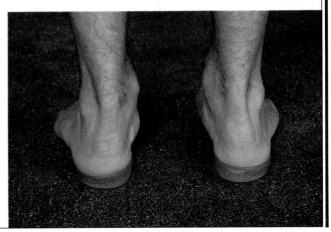

Straightened by new orthotic inserts, the patient's feet show instant improvement: The devices have raised the inner edges of the heels; body weight thus is shifted to the center of each foot. The patient will wear the orthotics in his ordinary shoes.

these inherited conditions can be diagnosed at home. Wet your foot so that it will make a footprint on a sheet of paper. If the entire outline of your foot is revealed, you have a low arch—a so-called fallen arch or flat foot. If most of the foot is visible but with a small area scooped out at the side, the arch is normal. If the print shows only heel and toe areas connected by a thin side strip, the arch is high. Although arch defects become evident in bone structure, their underlying cause may be with the muscles connecting ligaments that hold the arch assembly together. If those muscles are too flabby, the arch flattens; if they are too tight, it rises.

When flat feet cause pain, they do so because they cannot distribute the forces of walking and standing straight between the heel and ball of the foot. The pronating motion that every foot goes through in walking—flexing downward and rolling toward the inside as it is set down on the ground—becomes exaggerated, and the foot begins to collapse inward. The arch is still there, but it has leaned over, so that the victim of overpronation walks virtually on the inside of his foot. This twisting pulls on the muscles and ligaments of the foot, making them sore.

The handicaps of flat feet have been exaggerated. Many famous runners, including the great Olympic sprinter Jesse Owens, had flat feet. And although the United States Army rejected flat-footed men in World War I, it accepted them for combat duty in World War II.

The troubles caused by flat feet can be alleviated through exercises, such as stretching the calf muscles or rising up and down on the toes, that strengthen muscles and ligaments in the foot. Small wedge-shaped inserts in the shoe, or orthotics *(pages 77-79),* may help to make sure the heel strikes correctly and keep the arch from leaning over. However, such arch supports should be used only at the direction of a doctor; store-bought inserts purchased on the hunch that they might help correct overpronating feet may do the opposite and allow muscles to relax that should be encouraged to work on their own again.

Oddly enough, while flat feet attract attention, an arch that is too pronounced generally escapes notice; it can actually cause more discomfort. It is high partly because taut ligaments keep it so, pulling on the tarsal bones and holding them rigid. The steep angle of the arch pushes down on the ball of the foot and the arch does not flex to absorb shock. Cushiony soles can make up for the arch's rigidity, and an arch support can redistribute this painful concentration of pressure. But often the main difficulty with a high arch is finding shoes that fit: Those that seem all right in the toe and heel may be hard to lace, while those that can be laced easily may be too long.

Easing foot strain

The ligaments that may make arches high or low are also at the root of simple foot strain, the tired, aching feeling that plagues everyone at one time or another. This can result from any out-of-the-ordinary activity that puts excessive stress on the ligaments. The vacationer who takes a 10-mile hike on the first day in the country, the ordinarily sedentary party-goer who dances with unaccustomed vigor into the night, the office worker who walks all the way home on her high heels

Foot doctor to the world

The miseries of flat feet were well known to turn-of-the-century Chicago shoe salesman William Scholl: He heard about them from customers every day. At the time, the best available remedy was simple rubber wedges that were placed under each foot's arch, acting as little more than a cushion inside the shoe. But Scholl, a gifted tinkerer, invented something better: a comfortable leather-sheathed ridge made of opposing plates of springy metal. Placed in the shoe, it boosted the drooping arch and flexed slightly as the wearer walked.

The arch support was an immediate success. Scholl, whose shoe-selling talents meantime had helped him pay his way through medical school, quickly formed a company—still known by his name—to make and sell the device. In the ensuing decades, Dr. Scholl developed dozens of foot-care products; his keen appreciation for advertising is revealed in the memorabilia at right.

Dr. William Scholl demonstrates the fit of one of his newfangled arch supports in this studio photograph taken in 1904.

because it is such a lovely evening—all are using their feet abnormally, and their feet will probably hurt. But the postal worker who must pound hard pavements for months on end, the repairman who must constantly squat on the balls of his feet and the jogger who regularly thumps his way through mile after mile may also suffer strain, though it develops over a longer period of time.

Repeated contracting of certain muscles while others are less severely taxed can create an imbalance that will put extra stress on the ligaments, and they become inflamed. The pain can occur in several spots, but the principal target is the plantar fascia along the sole; any place along it—under the entire length of the arch—can hurt.

The remedy is simple. Massage the foot and soak it in warm water. The pain should go away after a day or two. To prevent recurrence, exercise; rising up and down on the balls of the feet increases the flexibility of ligaments and strengthens muscles. One jogger who nursed vague arch pains for a

year and a half began doing such exercises and found his aches gone in a couple of days.

Although foot strain cannot always be avoided, common-sense measures can prevent the worst aches. For one thing, wear shoes that fit the occasion and the surface. Running shoes designed for jogging on grass or a cinder track will not protect adequately on concrete or asphalt. For long sightseeing walks in cities, fairly thick soles and substantial arch support help. For hiking in rough country, heavy soles protect the arch, and tops that lace up over the ankle provide extra support. Perhaps the most tiring activity of all is simply standing still in one place; sturdy shoes help, but greater aid is provided by movement: Shift weight from one foot to the other and walk around, even if only for a few steps.

Such care should be all that is necessary to keep the feet in good condition. Their burden is unique, but so is their structure. Given knowledgeable attention, they will serve their owner well.   ❄

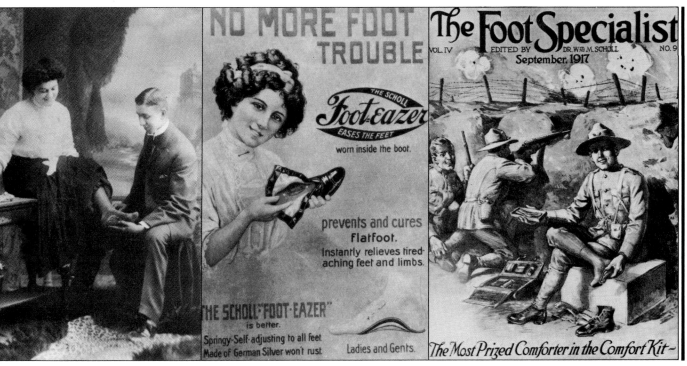

A display card touts Dr. Scholl's first successful invention—"foot-eazer" arch supports. They sold for two dollars a pair. In 1907, Dr. Scholl invented corn pads: molded-rubber cups, held in place by adhesive, that loosened the painful growths.

While his comrades fight on in the trench beside him, a beaming doughboy takes comfort from a Scholl support. This fanciful World War I scene graced a 1917 cover of The Foot Specialist, a magazine for shoe retailers edited by Dr. Scholl.

CHAPTER 4

How to take care of sprains and strains

Charley horse and slot-machine tendinitis
Defending against tennis elbow
Intense, random pain from bursitis
Treating yourself with RICE
The drugs: more than painkillers
For relief—wet heat
Quick repairs through surgery

Sprains and strains are the most common miseries that afflict the human frame. They include a host of ailments ranging from twisted ankles to wrenched knees, tennis elbow and bursitis-stiffened shoulders; they generally strike some part of a joint, harming the ligaments that hold it together, the muscles or muscle tendons that move it or the various cushions that smooth the motions of all these parts. They confuse even doctors, for the major symptom is pain and it may be caused by any of many different kinds of injury, all difficult to diagnose. Incorrect diagnoses are frequent.

Fortunately, many sprains and strains can be prevented by common-sense attention to fitness, along with the proper shoes or athletic gear. And when these injuries occur, most not only cure themselves, but get better faster if very simple home remedies are applied at the right time.

Still, a doctor's advice may be needed to confirm the adequacy of home treatment, for some afflictions of this type do not heal readily. If treatment of them is delayed or misguided, the consequences can be serious. Said the British orthopedic surgeon, Sir Reginald Watson-Jones, "It is worse to sprain an ankle than to break it."

Not everyone knows the proper treatment for a sprain. Too many people, confronted with a twisted ankle, either plunge it into warm water or try to walk it off, or both. But heat, unlike cold, encourages blood flow and promotes swelling, while walking it off risks grave complications.

Part of the confusion comes from the similarity between two words, strain and sprain, and the frequent difficulty of distinguishing one disorder from the other. Knowing what they are and how they can occur may enable you to decide whether or not you can deal with them on your own.

A strain is any damage to a muscle, or to the tendon anchoring a muscle, that generates pain; it is what you feel when you strenuously exert a muscle that is not accustomed to heavy demands, as when you are painting a ceiling, carrying a heavy suitcase or engaging in an active sport without adequate preparation. The muscle's connecting fibers may be pulled unduly, or inflamed, or even slightly torn. Strains sometimes lead to complications, such as bursitis, involving adjacent tissues. They almost always afflict areas near a joint, but not inside it. And strained muscles or tendons will almost certainly repair themselves if given a period of rest without further aggravation.

A sprain, by contrast, is damage to the ligaments, the connectors that bind up joints. It occurs when ligaments are partially or completely torn, and the harm is usually done through an accident or because of a sudden blow of the kind often suffered in sports.

A sprain is generally more dangerous than a strain. Any weakening or failure of a ligament may cause further damage by leaving the joint improperly aligned, endangering other parts of the joint such as cartilage. A sprain also generally takes longer to heal. Sometimes a strain will lead to or even directly cause a sprain, as when a strained and weakened muscle is unable to move limbs properly and thus imposes extra stress on a joint such as the knee. Severe sprains are

His body parallel to the floor, his arms and shoulders generating some 300 pounds of force—more than double his weight—sinewy American gymnast Kurt Thomas works out on rings. To avoid the sprains and strains that this demanding routine might cause, Thomas does gentle flexibility exercises beforehand.

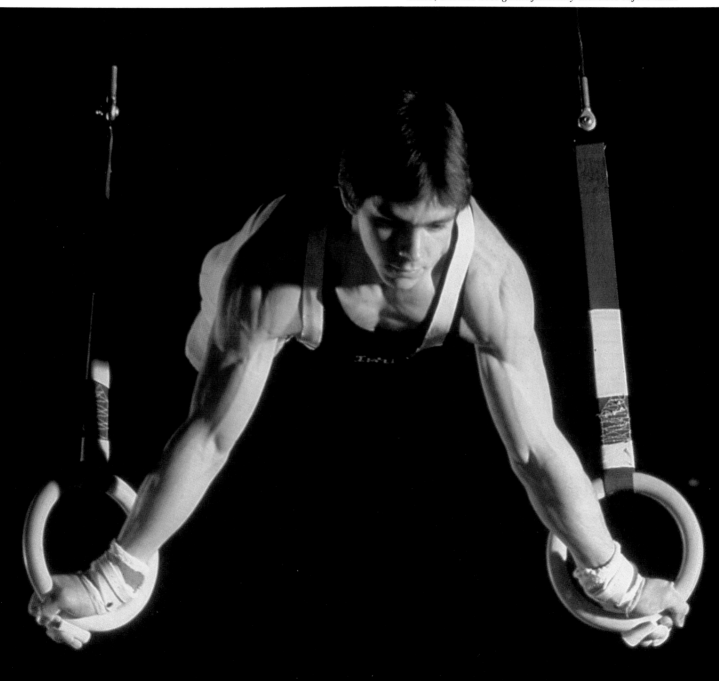

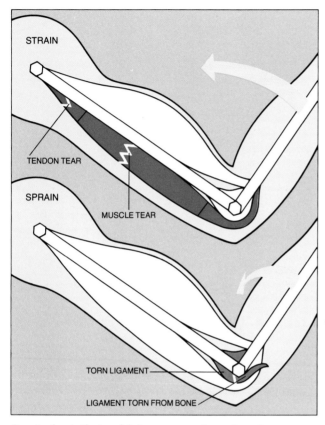

STRAIN

TENDON TEAR

SPRAIN

MUSCLE TEAR

TORN LIGAMENT

LIGAMENT TORN FROM BONE

Despite the similarity of their names, strains and sprains are different injuries with different causes. A strain results when either muscles or tendons (red)—the tough tapered muscle tips connected to bone—are stretched too far and tear. A sprain is caused by twisting that rips loose or tears ligaments (blue), the fibrous bands connecting bones.

often difficult to distinguish from fractures—the doctor must order an X-ray to know for sure.

Although any joint can be sprained, some are more vulnerable than others. The most vulnerable of all is the ankle. Sprained ankles have become one of the more common problems treated in emergency clinics. The injury is so debilitating that professional football teams in America use some 5,500 miles of tape each season in an attempt to protect their stars' ankles. Sprained ankles are also the special bane of weekend athletes, sending rock climbers, hikers and skaters to the hospital in huge numbers.

Why the ankle is vulnerable

Although it is narrow and fragile, the ankle is called upon to support a great deal of weight while it is flexing, extending and twisting. Under particular stress are the ligaments on the sides, which have the job of linking the ankle knobs—those bony protuberances of the lower ends of the leg bones—to the foot bones beneath.

The ligaments on the inner side of the ankle are somewhat stronger than their single counterpart on the outer side. Not surprisingly, then, it is the weaker, outside one—the anterior talofibular, which projects forward from the ankle bone to secure it to the heel—that gives way more often. Most ankle injuries are so-called inversion sprains, in which the bottom of the foot inverts, or turns inward. This turn overstretches the anterior talofibular and can tear it.

Because the great majority of sprained ankles result from inward twists of the foot, the obvious way to prevent them is some artificial restriction on this movement of the joint: a shoe or tape that ties foot and tibia—the larger of the two lower-leg bones—together so that one cannot turn very far sideways relative to the other.

Taping will limit motion and increase stability of the ankle if it is done properly and remains tight. But even when tape is put on tight, it may loosen more than 75 per cent during vigorous activity.

Somewhat less stability is provided by high-topped shoes —the higher the top the more firmly it limits sideways twists. Rather rigid, high-topped boots have always been used to protect the ankles in hiking over rough terrain, and they are obviously necessary for skiing, to transmit movements of the hips and the upper legs to the skis.

Protection in strong muscles, supple ligaments

But the best protection against a sprained ankle is not equipment but the muscles and ligaments themselves. All of the leg, not just the ankle, must be developed. There are various exercises that will do this. To strengthen the calves, repeatedly stand on tiptoe, then lower your body to stand with heels on the ground. For muscles along the front of the legs, kneel down with your toes straight back and gently sit back on your heels, pressing the top of your feet downward to the ground. Hamstrings, the ligaments at the back of the thigh, will be stretched if you sit on the floor with your legs spread and bend forward to touch and hold each foot with both hands. To stretch the quadriceps, at the front of the thigh, first lie on your side, then bend the uppermost knee, grab your ankle with your outstretched arm and pull the ankle straight back until you feel resistance in the thigh.

Some very simple exercises can develop all three parts of the leg at once. For example, walking in water up to your waist—the shallow end of a swimming pool—provides good resistance against which to strengthen the quadriceps, calf and hamstring muscles.

Such exercises will increase both strength and flexibility of muscles and ligaments. Too much flexibility in the ankle ligaments, however, can make the joint so loose that sprains there become more rather than less likely. To develop approximately the right amount of ankle flexibility, exercise by moving the joint through each of its four normal motions: Slowly move your foot as far as you can comfortably up and down several times, then inward and outward.

Although the ankle is the most frequently sprained part of the body, it has the advantage of succumbing in a fairly straightforward manner: The sprains that befall it are all more or less the same. No such simplicity can be claimed by the knee, which is the largest and one of the most complex joints in the body, with its own maze of interwoven muscles, ligaments and other tissues. Moreover, the knee is frequently called upon to absorb pressures and execute maneuvers for which it does not seem to be designed.

The principal task of the knee is flexing the leg, a motion used to step up or down and to smooth the action of walking. Sudden stops and starts can put such a load on the knee that its ligaments give way. It cannot handle much in the way of a sideways swing or a rotational twist. Yet it must absorb twisting stresses every time the body rotates from the hips—a motion most people perform slowly and gently but that athletes often do fast and hard. And a sideways blow—common in body-contact sports such as football but just as easily caused by a collision with a low table in a dark room—can result in severe damage to this joint. Athletic history is studded with career-stopping knee injuries to great players. Bobby Orr in hockey, Joe Namath in football, Pete Maravich in basketball—all had their playing days cut short by knee trouble. Even joggers are susceptible, if they pound the pavements too strenuously.

The knee joint connects the thighbone with the kneecap and with the tibia, the larger of the two lower-leg bones. (The other bone of the lower leg, the fibula, is attached to the tibia below the knee, outside the joint.) Holding the femur, tibia and kneecap together are five ligaments: two side ligaments, two that crisscross inside the joint and a fifth that comes down in front to tie the kneecap to the tibia.

Most blows that strike a knee are delivered from the outer side, thus bending the knee inward, toward the other knee, and stretching—or tearing—the inner ligament. Often the ligament will also pull loose other parts of the joint. Especially susceptible is the inner meniscus, one of the two cartilage-like cushions, somewhat similar to spinal discs, that fit between the ends of the femur and tibia and enable the joint to endure shocks. One meniscus is located on the inner side of the joint, between the bones, the other on the outer side, but only the one on the inner side is connected to a ligament. If the pulled ligament tears loose a piece of that meniscus, the knee joint is unbalanced and it may buckle or lock.

For a variety of reasons, the other joints are not sprained nearly so often as the ankle and knee. The hip has exceptionally strong ligaments, connecting bones whose motions are

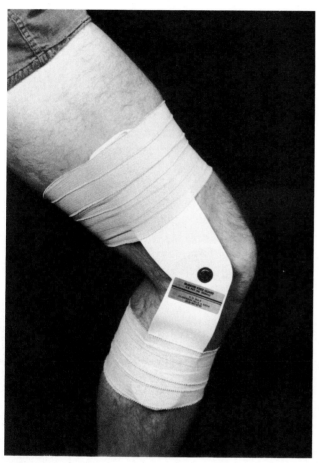

A hinged plastic knee brace weighing only eight ounces lets the victim of a sprained knee walk—and even play football—while the joint's torn ligaments heal. Taped to the leg, it shores up the weakened joint, supporting the wearer's weight, and buffers broadside blows that might cause further harm.

somewhat limited. The wrist and elbow rarely support body weight and so are less exposed to sprains. The shoulder, the most maneuverable joint in the body, is so loose and flexible that its ligaments are quite slack. What keeps it from coming apart more often than it does is not these ligaments but the many strong muscles and tendons that surround it.

Charley horse and slot-machine tendinitis

Any muscle and its connected tendons—from the toes to the back of the head—can be strained, and the strains can arise in so many distinctive ways that most have acquired special names. Some names suggest the circumstances of the injury (swimmer's cramp, slot-machine tendinitis), others identify the area of the body afflicted (shin splints), and a few are simply colorful nicknames (Charley horse).

No one really knows why a strain of the quadriceps muscle at the front of the thigh is called a Charley horse. The injury is one example of a broad class of strain, the cramp. Cramps are caused by sudden and excessive demands on a little-used muscle, which may rebel by going into painful, involuntary and sustained contractions.

Although a cramp is usually mild enough to produce only annoyance, it often prevents use of the muscle affected, and in rare cases it can be so severe it breaks a bone. One variety—swimmer's cramp—has been enveloped in a mystique that only now is beginning to be dispelled. Since great-grandmother's time this severe strain has been the subject of dire warnings to youngsters at the beach. It does sometimes pose a danger, for if a swimmer gets a cramp in his abdominal muscles he may be so disabled that he has difficulty reaching shore safely. But such cramps are infrequent. Cramps in the foot or calf muscles also affect swimmers; they can be alleviated by massaging the immobilized muscle while floating—an almost instinctive reaction.

Great-grandmother's prescription for preventing swimmer's cramp—do not go into the water until at least an hour after eating—is also in question. This caution was derived from the fact that, after a meal, stomach muscles demand oxygen to digest food. It was assumed that urgently needed oxygen supplies would be diverted from the muscles used for swimming; these muscles would be starved and a cramp would result. This idea, accepted as gospel for generations and printed in many otherwise-authoritative books, is not backed by any scientific evidence. It is no longer included in the protective advice provided by the American Red Cross. Most experts now believe that food has little, if any, connection with swimmer's cramp, which seems to be caused simply by fatigue or severe exertion.

Another type of strain with potentially serious complications is the whiplash injury that has become almost synonymous with rear-end automobile collisions (although it can also be caused by a stumble that pitches the body sharply forward). Two opposing sets of neck muscles are involved. One in front is overextended as the head suddenly snaps back all the way to the shoulder blades; then the other is strained as the head whips forward just as violently.

Whiplash occurs because humans have heavy, protective skulls and relatively weak muscles in the neck. According to Dr. Ayub K. Ommaya, a neurosurgeon at George Washington University Hospital, the human skull usually remains intact even after bouncing off a car's windshield. But the movement strains the supporting muscles, ligaments and joints in the neck.

Whiplash is a preventable injury, but not everyone tries hard enough to prevent it. Since 1969 cars have been equipped with head supports. "Quite often," noted Dr. Ommaya, "such headrests are too low, coming up only to the rider's neck." In that position the headrest cannot prevent the head from snapping back. His prescription: Position your headrest so that it touches your skull when your head is back.

Two strains that afflict athletes, shin splints and pulled hamstrings, also involve opposing sets of muscles. A shin splint, a strained muscle at the front of the lower leg, is often caused by unequal strength between the relatively weak shin muscles and the powerful calf muscles at the back of the lower leg. Some authorities believe that a pulled hamstring is due to an imbalance between the hamstring, at the back of the thigh, and the opposing quadriceps muscle at the front. From his tests of runners, however, Lee Burkett, Director of the Human Performance Laboratory at Arizona State University,

became convinced that the injury is traceable to an imbalance between the quadriceps of the left thigh and that of the right. He found that subjects with more than a 10 per cent difference in strength between these two muscles were subject to a greater risk of hamstring pulls. Both of these strains are readily prevented by the same strengthening exercises recommended for avoiding a sprained ankle.

More common among active, muscular people than muscle strain—and more painful—is strain of a tendon, or tendinitis. Individuals in good physical condition are particularly vulnerable because their muscles, strengthened by exercise, increase the tension on the relatively inelastic tendons. When tendons are tensed, they can rub against bones, ligaments and other tendons, tearing slightly. This irritation inflames the tendon or its sheath, resulting in tenderness and sometimes excruciating pain.

Tendinitis is insidious because it can seem to cure itself without really doing so. The pain may abate when the muscle is used, so the sufferer uses it—and risks a repeat. Many an athlete, wrote Dr. Don O'Donoghue of the University of Oklahoma, "goes right back to performing the same thing that caused the problem in the first place."

Defending against tennis elbow

Perhaps the most common form of tendinitis is tennis elbow, which at one time or another affects perhaps half of the estimated 30 million amateur players in the United States, as well as countless millions who do not play tennis but whose occupations or hobbies require forceful bending of the arm: politicians shaking hands on the campaign trail, crew members pulling their oars, carpenters and mechanics who must swing hammers and wrenches. At least one physician has developed tennis elbow from the snapping motion of resetting his fever thermometer, and more than one executive has developed the affliction from carrying a heavily loaded briefcase.

When the origin of tennis elbow is tennis, the ailment is usually caused by incorrectly executed backhand strokes, which overstress the forearm muscles used to bend the wrist up. That stress is transferred to the tendon that anchors the muscles to the bony knob on the outer side of the elbow.

A less common variety of tennis elbow, involving the muscles that are used to bend the wrist downward, affects the tendon anchored to the protuberance on the inner side of the elbow joint. This particular variety of tennis elbow is usually caused by the sudden wrist snaps that are used by professional tennis players in booming serves, and also by golfers who are following through with their stroke at the end of a powerful drive.

The best defense against tennis elbow, whether it stems from tennis or carpentry, is strong and well-stretched muscles in your forearm. Simple weight-lifting routines serve well. All you need are some five-to-10-pound dumbbells or other weights that can be easily held in one hand. Lay your arm flat on a table, palm downward, with your hand and wrist extending over the edge of the table. Holding the weight, bend your wrist up and down 10 times. Turn your arm over so that it is palm up, and repeat the exercise. Increase the number of repetitions to 15 as your wrist and forearm strengthen; alternatively, start with a lighter weight and work up to 10 pounds when you can perform 10 or more repetitions without experiencing pain.

Sports and exercise activities other than tennis have their own characteristic sites for tendinitis. In jogging, the strain-prone spot is the tendon that anchors the calf muscle to the heel, the Achilles' tendon, named after the mythological Greek warrior whose body was invulnerable to harm except at the heel. If the calf muscles are very tight and inflexible, as they may be in someone who runs great distances, the Achilles' tendon may strain until it snaps with an audible pop. More often, however, strain results in inflammation and tenderness that make running, or even walking, very painful.

Anyone undertaking an exercise that requires much running, such as jogging, should also make a special effort to prevent injury to the Achilles' tendon by keeping the tendon supple: Stretch it by standing barefoot about two feet from a wall and leaning forward with your back straight and your heels on the ground. Hold that position for 20 or 30 seconds, then return to an upright position. Repeat four or five times morning, afternoon and night. Shoes are important, too, for worn-down heels increase the likelihood of strain on the Achilles' tendon by throwing the foot off balance. If you feel tendinitis developing, check your shoe heel and replace or repair it if more than a quarter inch is worn away. If the heel is still good, or if you are using an athletic shoe with no heel, you can often prevent or relieve tendinitis with special orthopedic inserts that raise heel height inside the shoe.

The amount of stress any tendon can bear decreases with age, making some forms of tendinitis and related ailments common complaints after about age 30. The shoulder, by an anatomical quirk, is particularly vulnerable. One tendon anchors a shoulder muscle to the upper-arm bone, or humerus. In one form of tendinitis, each time the arm is raised that tendon is pinched between the bony surfaces of the humerus and the shoulder blade.

Such shoulder tendinitis most often develops following strenuous activities such as painting ceilings or chopping wood. But outbreaks of this ailment have also been reported among gamblers in the casinos of Lake Tahoe, Nevada. Slot-machine tendinitis, as it was dubbed by Dr. Richard Neiman, who investigated the phenomenon, produced extreme pain in the victims' right shoulders after the repeated strain of pulling the slot-machine levers. ''Optimal treatment,'' joked Dr. Neiman, ''is winning a jackpot early.''

Intense, random pain from bursitis

The elderly and the middle-aged are often victims of a complication of tendinitis that is also most common in the shoulder. Called bursitis, it is an inflammation of a bursa, one of the small, fluid-filled sacs named after a Greek wineskin of similar shape.

Normally, the body's 140 or so bursae act as cushions to reduce friction between tendons, ligaments and bones as they slide over or rub against one another. But after a tendon is injured, small quantities of calcium salts are deposited by blood at the site of injury as part of the body's natural recuperative process. For reasons that are still imperfectly understood, these salt deposits sometimes interfere with the cushioning action of the bursae, particularly in the shoulder, causing unbearable pain.

Because bursitis and tendinitis may be related, many cases are misdiagnosed. But the nature of the pain serves as a clue for telling them apart. Bursitis is characterized by brief attacks of intense pain, usually lasting for a few days and recurring at random intervals. The pain of tendinitis can be just as severe; it is also much more persistent.

Although the overwhelming number of bursitis attacks occur in the shoulder, the ailment may also develop in the thumb, hip, elbow or knee, particularly in front of the knee just below the kneecap. There a bursa lies under the skin to smooth the movement of the kneecap when the knee is bent, and it is easily injured. In the past, when servants spent a great deal of time kneeling to scrub floors, the ailment was known as housemaid's knee. Today, gardeners, plumbers and brick masons are among the most likely to suffer. And among young people who spend endless hours kneeling on surfboards waiting for the perfect wave, the ailment has acquired a modern name, surfer's knee.

The hip is the site of several variations of bursitis: hip pointer, and bowler's and golfer's hip. Hip pointer afflicts the bony protuberance of the pelvis, just a few inches below the waist, where muscles are attached. Because the muscles that pull the thigh to the side pass over this point, any muscle strain caused by sudden or repeated sideward steps—moves required in many sports—can harm the bursae there.

While the pain of hip pointer is localized on the surface of the thigh, pain deep within the hip probably indicates bowler's hip. In this case, the muscle that extends the leg on the side opposite the player's bowling arm—the leg that the bowler thrusts forward as he releases the ball—becomes weary from overuse. This is the iliopsoas muscle; it originates in the lower spine area, passes through the pelvis and, by way of its tendon, attaches to the inside front of the thighbone. The bursa there absorbs the unaccustomed stress and becomes inflamed.

Although both hip pointer and bowler's hip are brought on by sudden steps, a third kind of hip bursitis, golfer's hip, can occur even if the feet are firmly planted on the ground. It can afflict anyone who rotates his hips, as a golfer does during a swing. In this instance, the probability of pain is

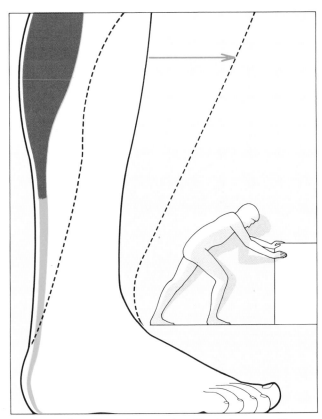

Connecting the calf muscle (orange) and heel, the vulnerable Achilles' tendon (yellow)—named for the mythological Greek warrior who was killed when an arrow pierced his unguarded heel—is easily strained when the leg pulls it in running (dashed lines). To make the tendon more resilient and so prevent injury, lean forward onto a support (right) and, keeping both heels on the ground, bend one knee until the calf muscle in the other leg feels noticeably taut. Hold the position about 20 seconds, then switch sides. Repeat the exercise three times.

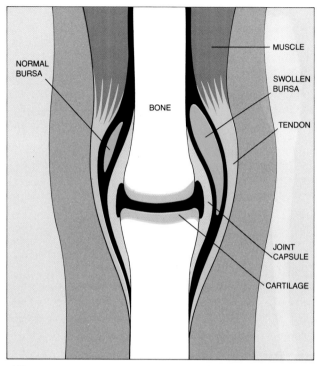

Adjacent to most joints are tiny sacs called bursae, which secrete fluid to ease friction between muscles, tendons and bones. Injury or constant pressure on bursae—from repeated kneeling, for instance—may cause swelling: bursitis. Unlike arthritis, bursitis seldom affects cartilage or other parts of the joint capsule —but the painful symptoms of the two diseases can be similar.

doubled: Both the hip pointer's bursa and the bursa of the iliopsoas muscle are affected by the stress of the unusual twisting motion.

Treating yourself with RICE

The main symptom of all strains and sprains is the same— pain on motion—and the initial treatment is the same, too. Indeed, for most of these injuries the initial treatment is all that is needed. Four basic elements are involved: rest, ice, compression and elevation, best remembered by the acronym RICE. Plus, of course, aspirin or acetaminophen.

In some cases the first part of self-treatment—staying still—may prove difficult. One Bostonian, having fallen while hiking alone down a New England peak, decided that her ankle was sprained and resolved to wait for help. Darkness came. All night long she sat stoically, even while a curious bear approached to examine her before wandering off. Her resolution was rewarded; in the morning, friends who had missed her came to the rescue. At the hospital, a doctor examined her ankle and confirmed the value of her patience; had she attempted to hobble off the mountain, she might have caused permanent injury to the sprained joint.

To rest an injured elbow or wrist, immobilize the arm in a sling. Slings are sold by most drugstores, but one can be improvised of any strong cloth. First, cut or tear a piece 42 inches square and fold it once to make a triangle. Then tie the two ends that are farthest apart in a knot, and slip the knot over the head and around the neck, putting the fold at the wrist and cradling the elbow in the corner, or right angle; let the sling extend an inch or so beyond the elbow. Adjust the remainder of the sling along the forearm so that the wrist and hand are supported; a dangling hand could place additional strain on the joint needing protection.

For the second ingredient in the RICE procedure, some form of cold is also almost always available—a bag of ice cubes, even a cold can of soda. Some first-aid kits include a lightweight chemical cold compress that remains inactive until it is needed; then the user breaks a small container inside the pack, and the resulting reaction produces cold that lasts for as long as half an hour.

The application of cold promotes comfort in several ways. First, ice acts as a local anesthetic, relieving the immediate pain of the injury. Second, ice slows or stops internal bleeding from the damaged tissues by forcing blood vessels to contract. This contraction counters the painful swelling, which is caused by blood from surrounding tissues leaking into the damaged area.

The third component of self-treatment, compression, also halts swelling. For injuries that break the skin and cause bleeding, the swelling may be useful, since it triggers the release of antibodies to fight infection. Most sprains and strains, however, leave the skin unbroken and there is no danger of infection; in these instances, the swelling of the joint simply retards the beginning of the healing process. To compress the injury, wrap an elastic bandage snugly, but not tightly, around it.

In applying both cold and compression, take care not to aggravate the injury. Elastic bandages provide only compression; they do not stabilize a joint enough to permit its use without risk of additional damage. And never apply ice directly to the skin, for the cold must be maintained so long that it may cause a cold burn; rather, place cubes or crushed ice in a plastic bag and wrap the bag in a towel. Every half hour remove the ice and unwrap the compression bandage to make sure that blood circulation is not impaired; after 15 minutes, reapply both bandage and ice.

The fourth element, elevation, is particularly useful in reducing the swelling of ankle and knee injuries. Elevation of the legs also serves as a reminder not to use the injured limb. Raising a hurt elbow or wrist above heart level helps reduce swelling because gravity then counters the pressure causing blood leakage. If it is impractical to keep the arm that high, a sling will help by reducing blood flow and preventing unnecessary movement, particularly the tossing and turning that often accompany sleep.

The drugs: more than painkillers

Aspirin is the only drug needed for minor sprains and strains; pain too great for aspirin to handle is one sign that a doctor's help is needed. He can prescribe more potent medications that, like aspirin, not only dull pain but counteract the cause of the pain, inflammation.

In addition to these generally accepted drugs there are a number of remarkably effective substances that are not recommended for mild or moderate pain because they may cause severe, possibly long-lasting side effects. Some of the potent anti-inflammation medications are synthetic steroids of the cortisone family, similar to the natural steroids that the body produces to control its internal defense system; they are prescribed for serious ailments such as arthritis *(Chapter 6)* but are usually considered too hazardous for routine use on strains and sprains. Still other drugs, such as DMSO (dimethyl sulfoxide) are potentially so hazardous that their use is in great dispute.

Aspirin is just one of a sizable family of anti-inflammation painkillers, most of which are available only by prescription. These drugs not only work in the same manner but also share an annoying side effect—stomach irritation, which may cause only a mild upset in most people but in some cases can precipitate peptic ulcers.

Ironically, aspirin's effect on the gastrointestinal tract is sometimes more severe than that of the related prescription medicines. Large doses of aspirin are often required to reduce inflammation, and about 40 per cent of all patients cannot tolerate such large amounts for prolonged periods. For them, prescription medicines such as ibuprofen, tolectin and ascriptin may act somewhat more gently on the gastrointestinal system.

Other anti-inflammation drugs such as indomethacin and phenylbutazone are very fast-acting and effective but introduce comparably bothersome side effects—not only stomach upset but skin rashes and headaches. Still others introduce reactions that are more serious yet.

Among the most powerful of the drugs in the aspirin family is phenylbutazone—generally known as bute. Synthesized in 1946, it quickly found wide use because it works very fast and very effectively, eliminating the pain and swelling caused by sprains and strains. It is extensively employed by sports trainers because it puts disabled players back into action on the field so promptly. And it is quite often prescribed by private physicians for nonathletic injuries—too often, in the opinion of many authorities, for it also introduces serious risks.

One hazard bute shares with other strong painkillers: Although it permits injured joints to work without hurting, the damaged tissues that have not healed can be permanently harmed by the vigorous activity. This effect has aroused criticism, even over the common practice of administering bute to race horses so that they feel better than they really are, which often causes the animal to put too much pressure on a bad joint. According to published reports, some horses dosed with phenylbutazone have run themselves to death.

For humans the serious reactions to the drug may include hepatitis, anemia and the retention of fluid in the body, an effect that can harm those suffering from kidney or heart diseases. Susceptibility to these actions increases with age, heightening the risk for the elderly. The entry on phenylbutazone medications in an official publication of the American Medical Association warns: "Generally they should be used only for brief periods."

Recent research has shed new light on the processes by which these drugs reduce inflammation and produce their less desirable effects. They counter the body's normal reaction to damage. When a ligament or tendon is injured, its bruised and torn blood vessels release a variety of substances that immediately go to work as if to fight infection. One of these is histamine, which stimulates the flow of blood while simultaneously dilating surrounding blood vessels, rendering them more permeable.

Through these now-porous vessels, blood fluids seep into the injured area, carrying a substance called fibrinogen, which forms clots, effectively sealing off the inflamed section and preventing the spread of bacteria or toxins. Strangely enough, all this busywork seems to be unnecessary for most sprains and strains. If the skin is not broken, there is no real danger of infection.

The inflammatory reaction runs its natural course unless interrupted by outside agents such as drugs or the application of ice. The duration and intensity of the reaction, scientists have now found, are regulated by substances called pros-

taglandins, which the body releases along with histamines.

It is the prostaglandins that are affected by aspirin and the related anti-inflammation drugs, but this was not realized until long after these remarkable body substances were discovered in the 1930s, by Swedish physiologist U. S. von Euler. He found them in human semen, noted that they could make muscle cells relax or contract and—mistakenly believing that they were present only in the male genital tract— named them after the prostate gland, which is located there. Today it is known that prostaglandins are present in almost every tissue in the body. They help regulate an enormous range of body functions, including the secretion of gastric acids in the stomach, the functioning of the kidneys and the contraction of muscles.

Prostaglandins affect the duration and intensity of inflammation by making blood vessels more sensitive to histamines and other chemicals. One of the effects of prostaglandins is to make blood vessels more permeable to the inflammation-producing fluids triggered by the histamines. If the release of prostaglandins is halted, the severity and duration of inflammation are reduced. In 1971, the pioneering research of Dr. John Vane and his associates at the Wellcome Research Laboratories in England demonstrated that aspirin and the aspirin-like drugs reduce inflammation by inhibiting the body's release of prostaglandins.

Researchers now believe that the suppression of prostaglandins by these drugs also leads to the drugs' gastrointestinal side effects, for the prostaglandins also regulate gastric acid. With fewer prostaglandins, inflammation is reduced, but excess stomach acid is released. A medicine that could suppress prostaglandins at the site of inflammation without simultaneously interfering with their regulatory functions elsewhere could reduce swelling and pain without creating stomach problems.

Prostaglandins themselves may play a key role in preventing the gastric side effects of such drugs. When prostaglandins are administered to laboratory animals by mouth or injection, these magical substances have prevented just the sort of gastric irritation caused by anti-inflammation drugs.

Important as the side effects of these aspirin-like drugs can be, they are less serious than the adverse reactions possible with the cortisone type of anti-inflammation agents, such as prednisone and prednisolone. The cortisone drugs also counter the body's natural reactions to injury but so powerfully that, when used for sprains and strains, they interrupt the normal healing process and can cause tissue degeneration in tendons and ligaments.

Despite their dangers, these medications are sometimes prescribed to achieve quick relief from intolerable pain of inflammation, particularly in severe cases of bursitis and tendinitis. Doses are generally limited to a maximum of two injections within a one-month period. Doctors familiar with the drugs' awesome power have coined a grim quip: When cortisone drugs are misused, they permit the patient to walk all the way to the autopsy room.

A liniment that dissolves inflammation

Disputes over possible side effects have also surrounded the quite different anti-inflammation agent, DMSO, since its first medical use in 1963. A clear, colorless and practically odorless liquid, DMSO was synthesized in 1866 by Dr. Alexander M. Saytzeff in the central Russian city of Kazan. Dr. Saytzeff noted some of the liquid's unusual properties— its drying effect on human tissue and its ability to dissolve almost everything he put in it—but his discovery was almost forgotten after his death. Then in the 1950s the chemical became available in large quantities as a by-product of the wood-pulp and paper industries, and it found a market as an industrial solvent. But its medical uses went unrecognized until an industrial chemist described its properties to Dr. Stanley Jacob, of the University of Oregon Medical School.

Dr. Jacob, who was searching for a way to preserve donated human organs for transplantation, was intrigued by the ability of DMSO to penetrate human tissue without apparent damage. In quick succession, he discovered an unprecedented range of medical applications for the compound. It penetrated rapidly into the bloodstream, either by itself or carrying other drugs or chemicals with it. It dried the skin, suggesting that it might be used in preventing infection of moist wounds in burn victims. Most amazing of all, DMSO

brought almost immediate relief from the pain and inflammation of sprained ankles and arthritic joints. To test other applications, and to study exactly how the magical substance worked, Dr. Jacob and numerous other investigators started clinical trials.

But the usual tests of new drugs, during which one group of volunteers receives a harmless, inactive substance and the other the drug under study, proved impossible to perform with DMSO. Within a few minutes of exposure to DMSO, volunteers developed an oysterlike taste in their mouths and a garlicky body odor that persisted for as long as 72 hours. These side effects were apparently harmless but they enabled the volunteers to distinguish between the DMSO and the inactive fake, and the mere fact that they could tell which medication they were getting influenced its effect on them, invalidating the tests.

In the interim, animal studies conducted by Dr. L. F. Rubin at the University of Pennsylvania indicated that DMSO caused eye damage in dogs. Dogs that had been given the chemical five days each week developed an abnormality of the lens after the ninth week. Later studies with rabbits produced similar results.

Out of fear that humans might suffer similar eye damage, most tests of DMSO were halted in the United States in 1965. By then, however, an estimated 100,000 Americans were already using the unproved and unapproved drug for regular treatment of sprains, strains and arthritis. Despite appeals and pressure to approve DMSO, federal authorities assented to its use for only one human application: a rare and painful bladder disorder. In addition, DMSO was approved for use on nonbreeding horses and dogs; on them the substance proved remarkably successful in relieving inflammation of sprains and bruises.

Veterinary and industrial stocks of DMSO soon supplied increasing numbers of people with DMSO. Eventually a few states permitted its sale for human use. The ban on tests of DMSO was only temporary, and later trials did not confirm the danger to human eyes.

Apparently DMSO works its cures so fast at least partly because it is such a powerful solvent. This characteristic

When to apply heat, when cold

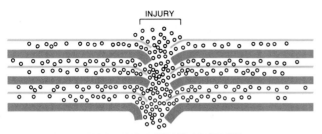

INJURY

TWO-STEP TREATMENT FOR A STRAIN OR SPRAIN
*Cold and heat are common prescriptions for hurt tissues (above)
of a sprain or strain, but which should be used? The answer is
both. When tissue is injured, inflammatory fluid (black circles)
seeps out around torn blood vessels (red) and nerves (green).
The damage is slowed by cold, then reversed by heat.*

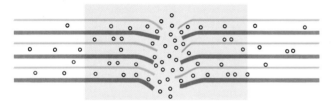

HOW COLD SLOWS SWELLING
*Cold packs should be applied immediately after injury and used off
and on for the first 24 to 72 hours, to reduce inflammation and
start recovery. The cold (blue) constricts swollen blood vessels,
restricting bleeding and fluid seepage. Cold also relieves pain
by reducing muscle spasms and slowing nerve impulses.*

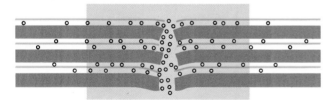

HOW HEAT SPEEDS HEALING
*After cold reduces inflammation, heat (peach) dilates blood
vessels to increase blood flow, bringing in nutrients and repair
agents such as scar-tissue cells and white blood cells that carry
debris away. Heat also accelerates chemical processes,
speeding the growth of cells to repair breaks in tissues.*

enables it to seep rapidly from the surface of the skin into the
bloodstream and thus travel to the site of an injury. There its
action may also depend on its power to dissolve other substances, for it seems to make the cortisone type of healing
agents more readily available to damaged tissues than they
otherwise would be. In addition, it may increase the infiltra-
tion of white blood cells that repair damage.

Concluded Dr. Harold Brown, a Seattle specialist in industrial medicine, who conducted trials of a DMSO gel:
"Eighty per cent DMSO gel is a safe and effective compound for the treatment of acute traumatic and inflammatory
musculoskeletal conditions—specifically, moderate and severe sprains and acute bursitis and tendinitis."

The results of Dr. Brown's study were confirmed by the
experimental use of DMSO on athletic injuries at Brigham
Young University, in Utah. Sports trainer Marv Robertson
said, "It gets to an injury quickly and enhances recovery. It is
not a healing drug. But if people accept it for what it is, I
think it is a breakthrough."

Robertson also pointed out that one of DMSO's most useful qualities, the speed with which it penetrates to an injury,
is also cause for concern. "It will take anything on the skin at
the time of application into the system," he warned. "So if
someone had been around a toxin and then applied DMSO to
an injury without washing, that toxin would be taken into the
system. That could be fatal."

Widespread, routine use of DMSO remains controversial.
The safety of the drug in high concentrations, in large
amounts or over long periods is yet to be affirmed by the
Food and Drug Administration. "The thing they're doing is
using an untested drug on young athletes," cautioned a government investigator, Roger Lowell. "What will that do to
that person in 20 years?" Until that question can be satisfac-
torily answered, the safest drug for sprains and strains
remains aspirin.

For relief—wet heat

After pain and swelling are eliminated, a sprain or strain is
ready for the final phase of self-treatment: heat applications
to stimulate blood flow to the damaged area. Heat relaxes

tensed muscles, stops muscle cramps and spasms, and increases blood flow.

It is generally best to wait six to 10 hours after the last ice treatment before applying heat; an abrupt switch from cold to heat could cause a resumption of the minor internal bleeding that was previously halted by the cold compresses. Any comfortable, readily available source of heat will do; wet heat is best. You might use a basin of warm water for a wrist or ankle, a warm shower for the shoulder or knee, or a hot-water bottle or electric heating pad used with a wet cloth for the hip or elbow (make sure the label on the electric pad says it is safe to use on the wet cloth). Another good method for applying wet heat is to soak a towel in warm water, wrap it around the injured joint, and then cover it with several layers of plastic wrap to hold in the heat and prevent dripping.

If heat applications cause a return of pain or inflammation, or if the pain and swelling do not subside after 24 hours or so, then it is time to see a doctor. Often a physician can diagnose a sprain merely on the basis of the patient's account of what happened (''I slipped on a pebble, fell down and right away felt pain on the outside of my ankle.''). In some cases he will order a special X-ray called an arthrogram, for which a dye is injected into the joint: The resulting picture will show not only whether or not a bone is fractured but the extent to which ligaments may be torn.

If no bones are broken and the damage is slight, the physician may simply tape the joint to provide firm support, and prescribe drugs and more rest and warm compresses. But if ligaments or cartilage are badly damaged, the doctor will either put the ankle in a cast, usually for four weeks, or advise surgery.

If the damage is not completely repaired when activity resumes, the action of the joint may be affected. Numberless victims who attempt to get up and around too soon, walking about on not-quite-restored limbs, end up with what is known as a trick joint. Some trick knees, whose ligaments have never regained full strength, buckle when subjected to any odd stress—when the owner is rushing for a taxi, or executing a new step on the dance floor. Other knees whose menisci have been damaged will suddenly lock as the injured menisci jam them, barring all movement temporarily. People so afflicted learn to unlock their pesky joints with shaking or stretching motions, or even by grasping their legs in their hands and coaxing the knee to move.

Quick repairs through surgery

Operations to remedy such defects of the joints once were rare because they required extensive surgery and long convalescence, but they are now done routinely, quickly and almost painlessly *(pages 96-107)*. Torn ligaments or tendons can be repaired or, if necessary, replaced with tissue transplanted from elsewhere in the joint. A substitute for such transplanted tissue has also been developed at New Jersey College of Medicine and Dentistry by Chief Orthopedic Surgeon Dr. Andrew B. Weiss. It is a strong filament of carbon that can be attached to the ends of severely damaged ligaments and tendons; the carbon acts as scaffolding on which newly developing tissue, naturally generated by the body, is guided into place. In time, the tissue surrounds the filament and toughens into a new tendon or ligament that is, in all respects, as strong and flexible as the original.

To repair a joint that has a damaged meniscus or torn cartilage, the surgeon merely removes the injured pieces; in many cases scar tissue will appear in its place and provide the needed cushioning. Such operations can now be performed with the pencil-sized arthroscope *(pages 100-101)*, which requires only small incisions, allowing speedy recovery. ''There is very little pain or discomfort,'' noted Dr. William Hamilton, orthopedic surgeon for the New York City Ballet. ''Most patients are able to walk the night of the operation without canes or crutches. There's no cast involved.'' One dancer was back performing just two weeks after a portion of her cartilage was removed.

For most people, however, recovery from a severe strain or sprain is not so fast. Even a minor injury calls for some follow-up attention—mainly exercise. The inflamed muscle, ligament or tendon needs time and exertion before it can regain its former strength. Then with further exercise, it will be stronger than it was before it was hurt, and much less likely to be hurt again. ✳

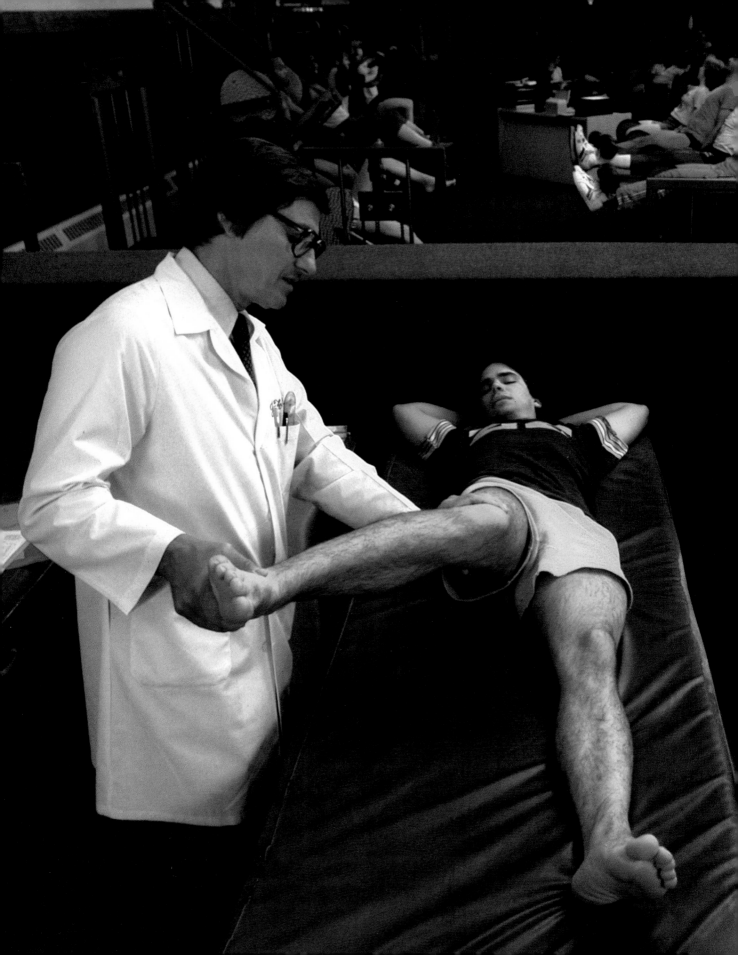

New ways to treat old woes

No longer need wrenching injuries to joints and muscles disable their victims for weeks or months at a time. Today most are quickly cured, thanks largely to treatments developed in caring for athletes. From clinics such as the Sports Medicine Center of the University of Pennsylvania in Philadelphia *(left and following pages)* have come techniques and procedures that are now used in hospitals around the world to mend the ankles and knees, elbows and shoulders that ordinary people hurt in everyday accidents.

The most notable of these advances in diagnosis, therapy and rehabilitation have come in the care of the knee, a joint that accounts for 60 per cent of the injuries treated at the Sports Medicine Center. The progress is due, in large part, to a single device—the arthroscope. Principally a viewing instrument, it is a slender, hollow metal probe up to six inches long that has a magnifying eyepiece at one end. The probe is inserted into the knee through an incision about a quarter of an inch long. Once inside the knee, the probe's fine strands of glass, or fiber optics, carry light into the joint, then conduct the reflections back and through the eyepiece, giving the doctor a clear view of the damaged tissue. "We can get right in there and look around for ourselves," said one enthusiastic physician. "There is no more guessing in knee surgery."

Although the scope's major advantage is its ability to provide, according to one physician, a "98 per cent precise diagnosis," it can play a key role in treatment as well. If the damage to the knee's internal structure *(below)* is not serious—a small tear, say, in the knee's cushiony cartilage—the view furnished by the arthroscope can guide the surgeon as he makes a repair. With arthroscope in place, he cuts other tiny incisions in the knee. Through them, he can insert delicate surgical implements and operate, snipping off and reshaping the damaged portions without cutting open the whole knee, as once was necessary. "You don't have the pain that you get with regular knee surgery," said one surgeon. Many of his patients are back on their feet and out of the hospital within 24 hours, a small bandage covering their incisions.

Whether the surgery is major or minor, any repaired joint must be rehabilitated exhaustively. Better understanding of the way stresses affect ligaments and muscles enables trainers or physical therapists to tailor exercise routines individually, depending on which tissues were injured, how seriously they were hurt and whether or not a limb or joint had to be immobilized for recuperation. For some exercises, specially designed machines *(pages 104-105)* control exertion, loading specific parts of the body in specific ways. But many others require no equipment other than a rubber ball *(page 103)*.

Manipulating a knee injured in touch football, Dr. Joseph Torg, director of the University of Pennsylvania's Sports Medicine Center, finds that it wobbles—a sign of ligament damage. The injury will require major surgery. After about four weeks' recuperation in a cast, the patient will begin rehabilitation, relying on exercises with weight machines such as those being used in the background.

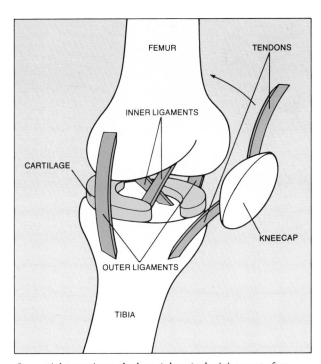

Once-tricky repairs to the knee (above), the joint most often hurt in sports, have now become routine. Most vulnerable are the cartilage crescents cushioning the contact between femur and tibia leg bones, and the inner ligaments, which are torn by frequently encountered sideways blows.

Getting a look at the problem

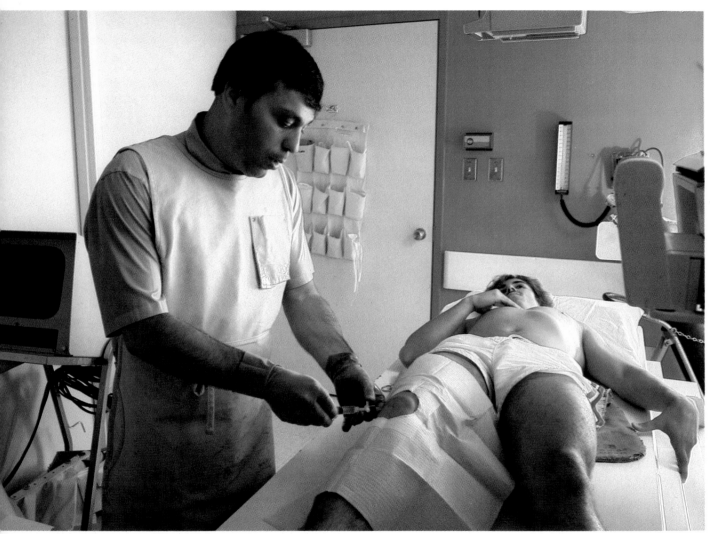

To X-ray soft tissues such as cartilage and ligaments, which ordinarily do not show up, Dr. Murray Dalinka withdraws fluid from a knee injured in soccer. He next will inject a dye that make soft tissues block X-rays, thus creating an image.

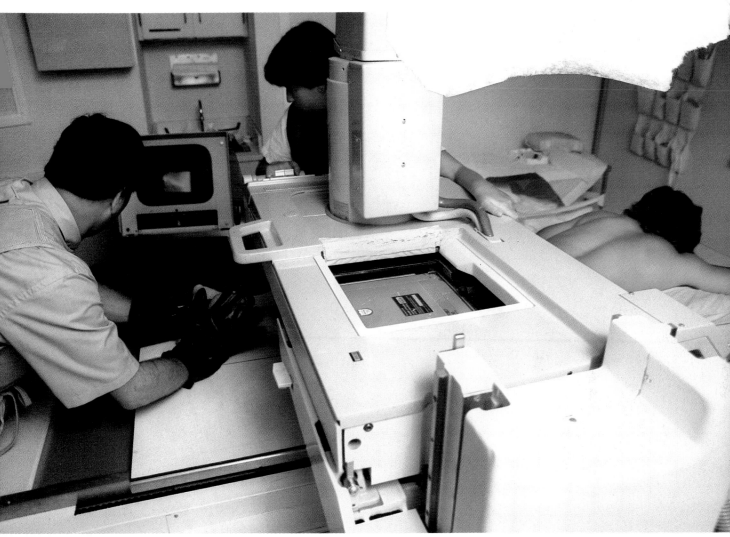

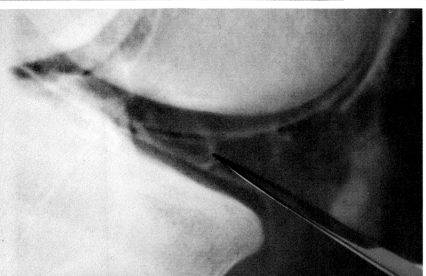

Lead-lined gloves protecting his hands against X-rays, Dr. Dalinka adjusts the wounded knee while he watches the video screen (left background). At left, one of the X-ray pictures he made reveals a tear in the knee's cushioning cartilage, visible as a white jagged line at the tip of the pointer.

Arthroscopy: surgery without scars

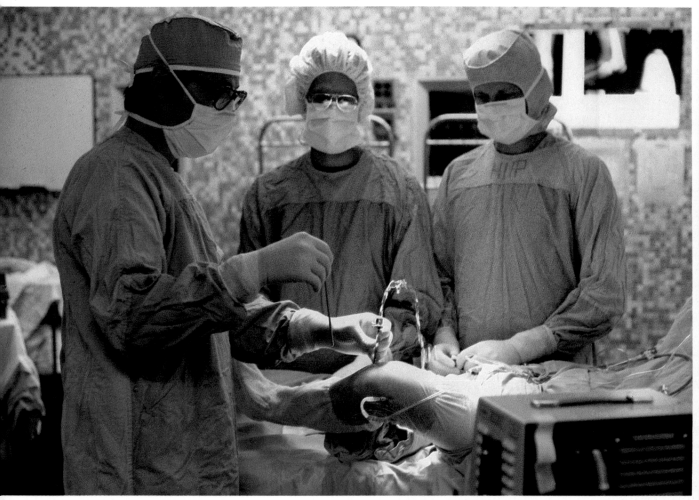

A salt solution injected into an injured knee squirts from an exit opening during an operation with an arthroscope. The device (in the surgeon's right hand) gives a view of the inside of the joint.

Only three small incisions were needed for this knee operation with an arthroscope: one for the viewer, another for the salt-solution tube and one for a shaver that cuts damaged tissue and sucks it out.

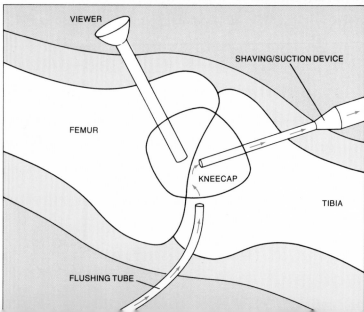

VIEWER

SHAVING/SUCTION DEVICE

FEMUR

KNEECAP

TIBIA

FLUSHING TUBE

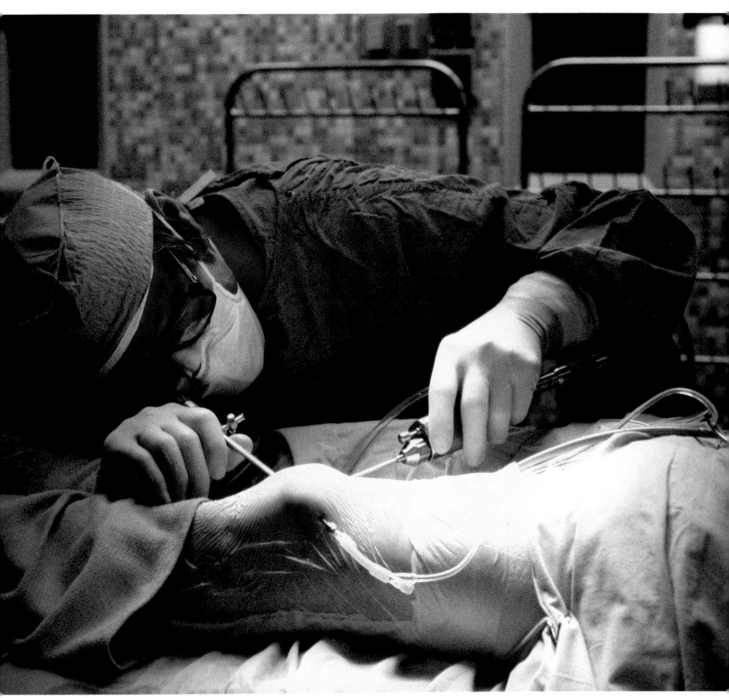

Watching through the arthroscope eyepiece, Dr. Torg with his left hand controls the shaver inserted into the knee to remove damaged cartilage. Unless removed, the torn cartilage flops around and causes more damage.

The path to full recovery

Ready to begin rehabilitation, Valerie Evans, whose knee cartilage and ligaments were repaired four weeks earlier, has her cast cut off with an electric saw by trainer Christine Bonci. The knee will be sensitive and stiff from disuse.

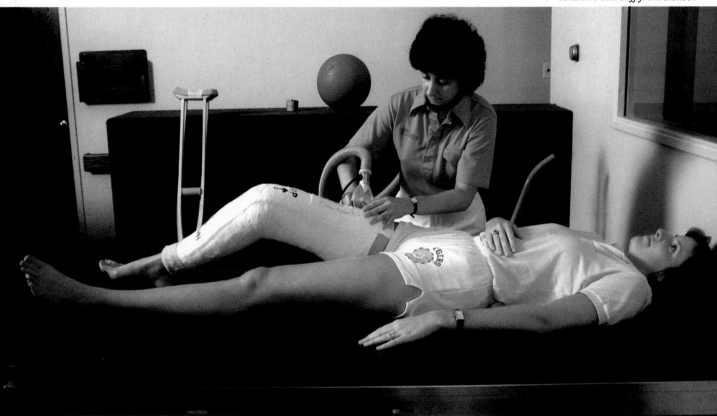

A "side leg lift" tones abductor muscles, which run from hip to knee on the outside of the leg—the first to weaken when the knee is immobile.

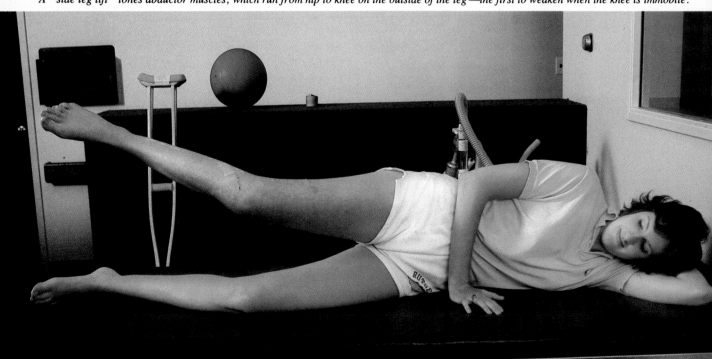

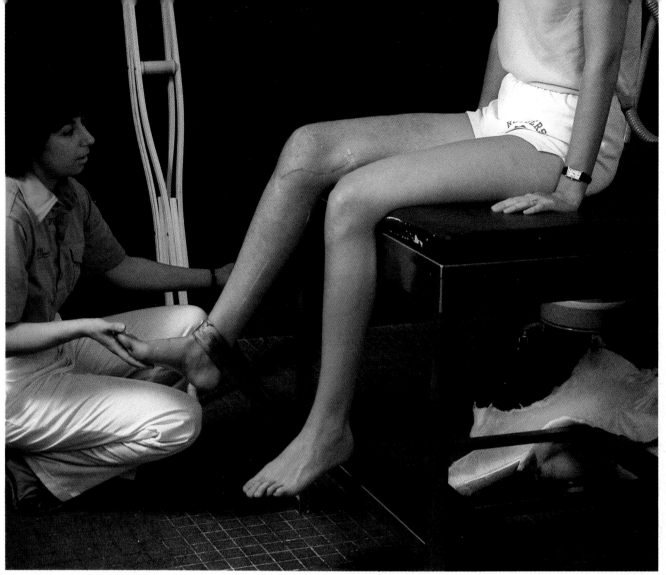

*Flexing her lower leg against a taut strap
while her trainer gently supports her foot,
Valerie Evans tries to extend her leg,
applying the maximum pain-free force for six
seconds; then she will rest and repeat
the exercise nine more times. This exercise
reconditions the quadriceps muscles
on the top of the thigh.*

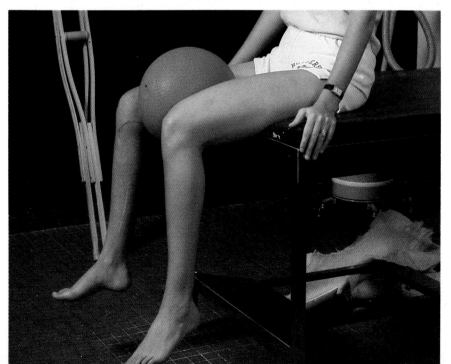

*Squeezing a large rubber ball between
the knees helps strengthen weakened groin
muscles. The patient presses her legs
together with all her might for six seconds,
and does that 10 times before proceeding
to more complex exercises.*

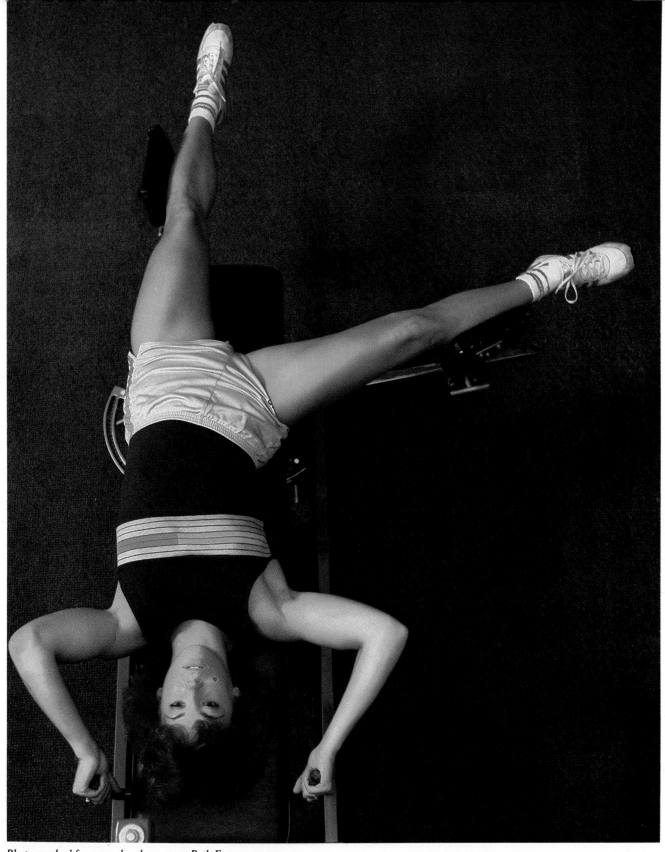

*Photographed from overhead, gymnast Beth Farnese uses a
weight machine to help rebuild a knee that was repaired by major
surgery a year earlier. While lying on the machine's padded
bench and grasping hand grips, she presses out with her injured
leg against resistance the device supplies; the exercise is
designed to strengthen abductor muscles.*

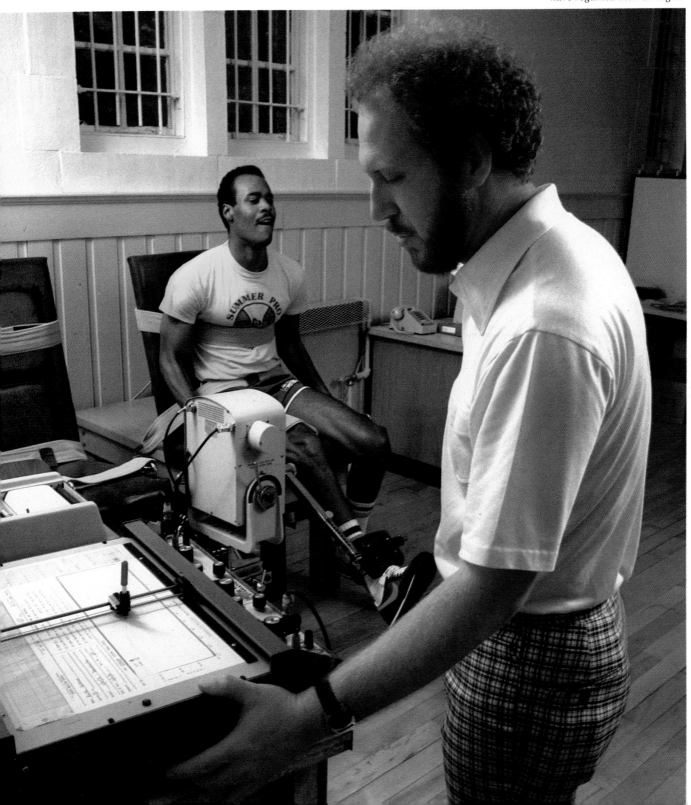

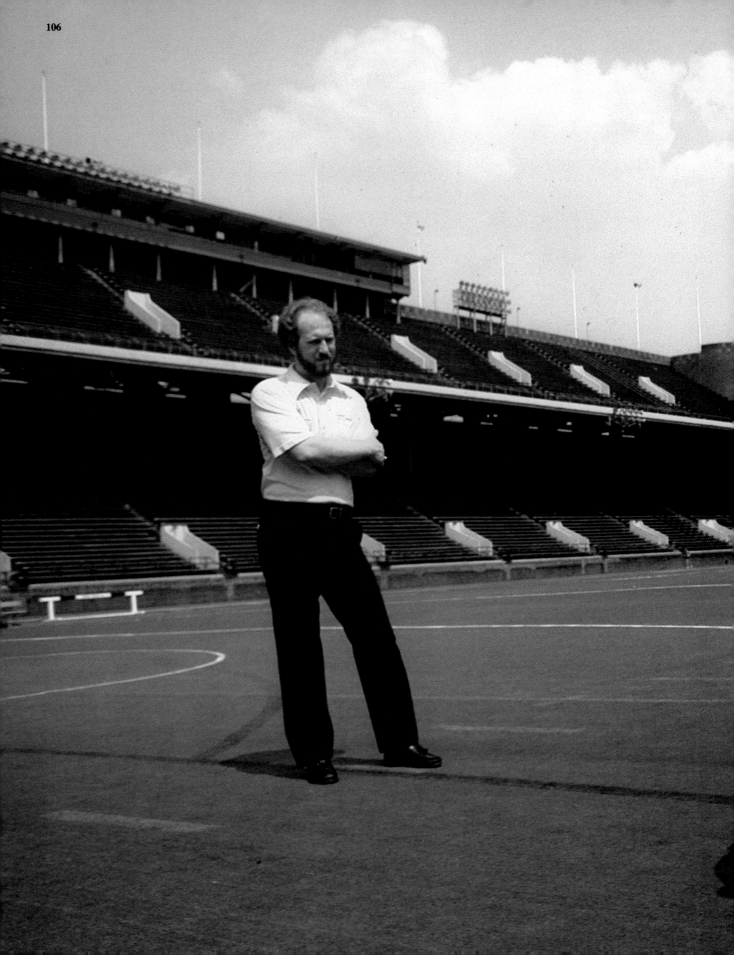

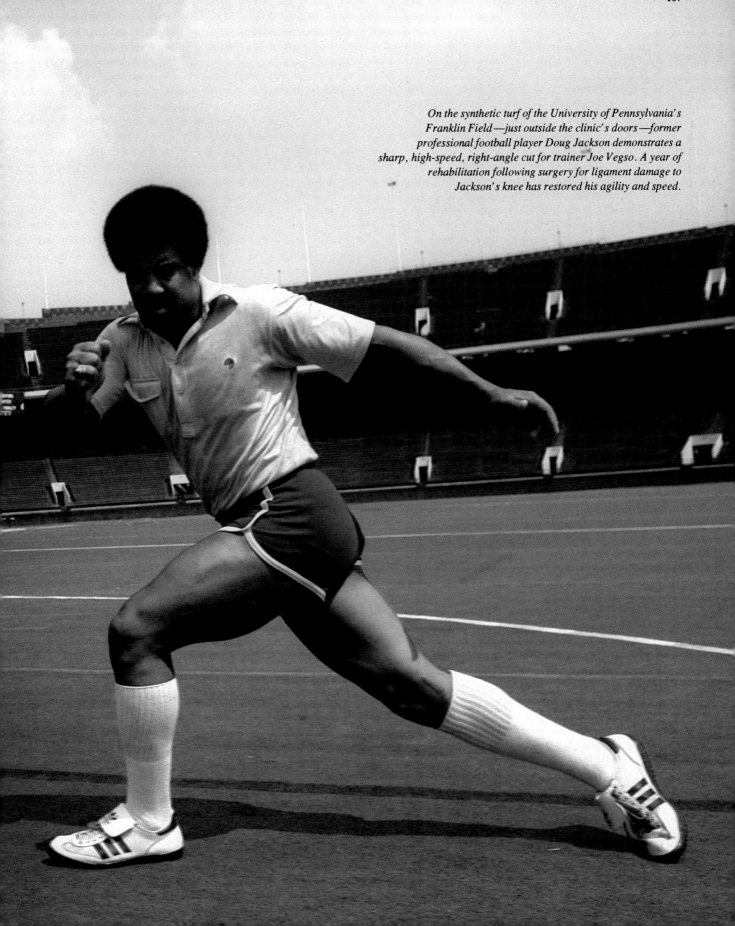

On the synthetic turf of the University of Pennsylvania's Franklin Field—just outside the clinic's doors—former professional football player Doug Jackson demonstrates a sharp, high-speed, right-angle cut for trainer Joe Vegso. A year of rehabilitation following surgery for ligament damage to Jackson's knee has restored his agility and speed.

CHAPTER 5

Working with nature to mend a break

The role of calcium
The fine art of reducing a fracture
Putting Humpty Dumpty together with man-made bone
For rapid recovery, keep active

Like most accidents, it happened suddenly. "I was up on a rickety stepladder, pruning a tangled wisteria vine," recalled the 58-year-old suburban New Yorker, "when I reached out too far and felt the ladder sway beneath me. Instinctively—I don't remember doing it—I put out my hands to break my fall, but as soon as I hit the ground I saw that I'd done something terrible to my wrists."

Even as the victim—a writer on medicine—lay on the ground and cursed his carelessness, he knew his own body was already racing to his rescue, as it began the miraculous business of rebuilding broken bone. His wrists became stiff and were swelling rapidly: The stiffness meant his muscles were going into spasm, contracting strongly to provide a kind of natural splint, while the swelling signaled blood rushing to the scene to begin healing. The blood would soon form a clot around the break, to be transformed in due course into a bridge linking the sundered parts.

Because this unlucky victim knew something about bone injuries, he was quite sure from the moment he hit the ground that he had suffered a break—a fracture—and not a dislocation, in which the end of a bone is knocked out of its natural position in a joint, tearing surrounding tissue in the process. But the two are not always easily distinguished.

The same kind of accident can produce either injury, and either is likely to distort the anatomy. A dislocation may appear easier to fix, but that is misleading. A dislocated joint often looks as if something has simply "popped out." The overwhelming urge is to pop it back in—but such a move

could cause further damage, particularly, as is often the case, if part of the joint is broken.

The safest way to proceed is to immobilize the injured member by cushioning it with a pillow, and to get immediately to a hospital. If there is an open wound—sometimes a broken bone will pierce the skin—do not touch it other than to cover it lightly with a sterile compress or clean cloth. And if there is any suspicion that either the neck or the spine has been injured, the victim should not be moved at all, even to place a pillow under his head; any slight shift can cause incurable damage, perhaps paralysis. Call for professional help and wait until it arrives.

At the hospital, the doctor will take X-rays to determine the precise nature of the injury. If it is a dislocation, he will ease the straying bone back into its joint and may provide some kind of splint or sling to aid the healing of torn tissues. Most dislocations heal fully in a few weeks, although hips may take months.

Fractures are trickier to handle. To begin with, broken bones usually must first be set—the fragments brought together in proper alignment to ensure that the bone will be straight after it heals. Once set, the fragments must be immobilized so they will not be jarred apart before bone repairs itself—a process that takes about eight weeks for many fractures. In the not-so-distant past, one or both of these crucial steps might have been impossible if the break was a particularly extensive or complicated one. Today, thanks to a number of advances made since World War II, doctors have

In this computerized X-ray, which uses colors to contrast tissues of different densities, the white outlines of a woman's left arm bone highlight a jagged gap where the bone is fractured.

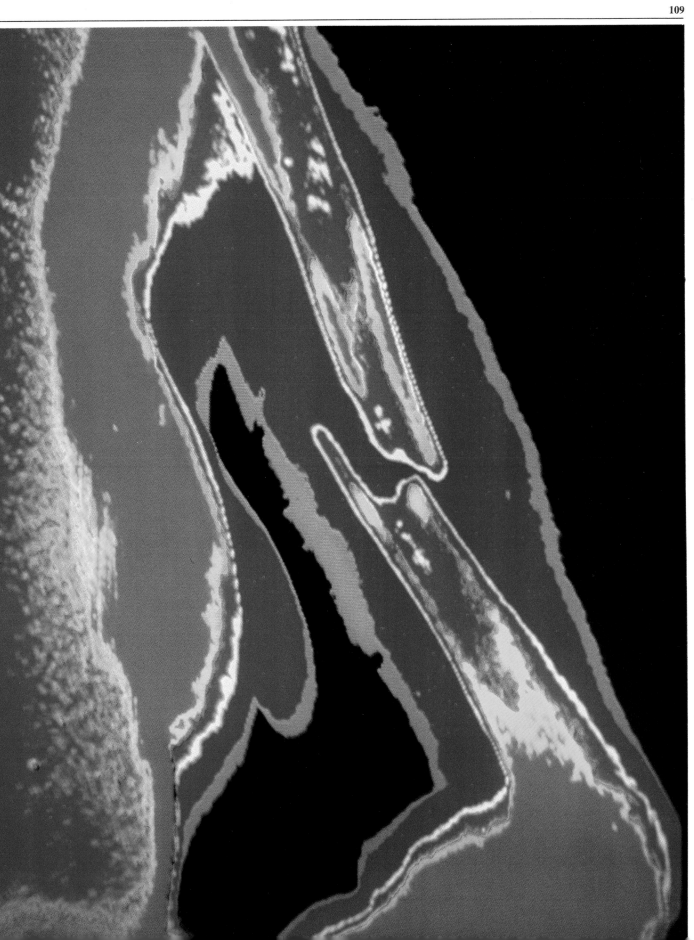

the tools and techniques to repair virtually any fracture.

Some of the new methods are refinements of old procedures. For example, patients suffering from breaks that do not show up on an X-ray can be injected with a special radioactive drug that is briefly absorbed into the bone, where it sends signals from the fracture site to a device called a bone scanner which then detects even the tiniest crack or chip. The character of casts has changed, too. Many people who once would have had to endure months in a cumbersome plaster cast—forgoing showers in order to keep it dry—can now have their broken limbs encased in lightweight fiberglass as tough as the hull of a speedboat and just as impervious to damage from water. Some children even go swimming with fiberglass casts, drying them later with a hair dryer.

The most important advances, however, have been in treating the fractures that used to result in disfigurement or disability. Badly fragmented bones, which in the past generally knitted themselves into misshapen, often unusable joints or limbs, can now be neatly pinned back together with surgically implanted wires, rods or screws, or held in position by pins or wires inserted directly through the skin. A bone so badly shattered that it cannot be reassembled at all may be patched with a spare part from elsewhere in the body, plastered over with a ground-bone paste or replaced entirely with a frozen bone taken from a cadaver. A crushed joint—which in the past would have permanently crippled its victim—can now be exchanged for a new assembly of plastic and metal.

Finally, the rare stubborn break that refuses to knit at all may be spurred into restorative action by electrical currents that encourage growth; this electrical stimulation has enabled people who once might have lost a limb or spent a lifetime on crutches to return to full mobility.

Such strides in treatment have made the repair of fractured bones less problematic and oftentimes less painful than ever before. This is good news indeed, for no matter how sophisticated the cures have become, no medical advance can eliminate the causes. Most fractures result from a sudden blow to part of the body—the arms, legs and collarbone are the most common sites—but bones can give way under all sorts of circumstances. Women have been known to suffer cracked ribs from too ardent an embrace. Some people, given a good scare, have snapped their heads so violently that the contracting muscle has pulled a piece of bone away from one of the neck vertebrae. The real wonder is that more people do not break their bones, because everyone flirts with fracture every day, whether by driving a car or walking downstairs or even opening a closet door in the dark.

Fashions in fractures

Certain fractures periodically come into style along with fashions in wearing apparel and fads in recreation. When high-platformed shoes were in vogue, orthopedists reported a sharp rise in the number of fractured ankles, as women lost their balance on the wobbly footwear. Fractures of the wrist, elbow and ankle appeared among roller skaters when adults rediscovered the childhood sport in the late 1970s. During the first nine months of 1979 alone, more than 17,000 roller skaters suffering such injuries limped or were carried into hospital emergency rooms in the United States.

When downhill skiing boomed after World War II, doctors encountered two characteristic leg fractures rarely seen before. The first was a spiral fracture of the tibia, caused by a fall on a leg corkscrewed by a twisting ski. The second was the so-called boot-top fracture, which occurs when a skier snags the edge of a ski, and the binding that holds the boot to the ski does not release. The lower leg, encased in the boot, comes to a sudden halt while the upper leg keeps going; both leg bones snap cleanly, producing a matched pair of transverse fractures four to six inches above the ankle.

However a person breaks a bone—whether in earning a living, in risky pursuit of fun or simply in slipping on a newly waxed floor—the severity of the fracture itself and the amount of time it takes to heal can vary enormously. For a variety of reasons, some people's bones are more resistant to damage and readier to mend than others'.

The single most important factor in determining whether or how a bone will break is age. Toddlers, although they fall down all the time in learning to walk, rarely break their rubbery, still-undeveloped bones. Older children generally suffer only hairline cracks or ''greenstick'' fractures: Their bones, like supple young twigs, bend and break partway through. However, an adult who falls heavily on a bone is likely to break it on impact. And a very elderly person may break a bone without striking it at all. Many old people who attribute a broken hip to a sudden fall have actually had the bone give way as they were walking down the street: The fracture caused the fall, not the other way around.

Fractures become more likely as the years pass because bones steadily become more brittle. But some adults unwittingly add to their risks. Obese people, for example, force their ordinary-sized skeletons to carry a larger-than-ordinary burden, taxing their bones with the stress. Sedentary people do not give their bones and muscles enough physical activity to trigger the vital remodeling process in which old bone material is continuously removed and replaced with new.

The most serious weakening of bones, however, is due to a puzzling process called osteoporosis, a degenerative bone disease that afflicts some 14 million elderly Americans. Osteoporosis is a progressive loss of bone material; bones become excessively porous and likely to break. The fact that four times as many women as men over the age of 50 suffer from osteoporosis indicates that hormonal changes at menopause play a part, but some of the blame can also be laid to bad eating practices and inactivity—habits that deprive the bones of the calcium and exercise they need for strength. Such inadequacies can harm even young people.

The role of calcium

Without sufficient calcium—most readily supplied by milk products—bones lack the materials they need for rebuilding. They can also lose much of the calcium they already contain. Several body systems—the muscles and the blood in particular—if deprived of calcium will turn to the handy skeletal storehouse for their needs, drawing the mineral directly from the bones.

A similar deficiency also can be caused by too much phosphorus. A diet rich in phosphorus—an element that is present in relatively large amounts in processed foods and soft drinks—tips the metabolic balance. Too much phosphorus increases production of a hormone that causes calcium to be

FIVE WAYS A BONE CAN BREAK
Bones, like any breakable objects, can separate or shatter in almost innumerable ways. But most fractures fit into one of five categories (below). The classifications are based on the appearance or direction of the fracture line. Any of these fractures may be either closed—if all damage is beneath the skin—or open, a potentially more serious break in which the skin is punctured by shards of bone and is susceptible to infection.

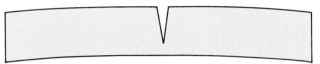

GREENSTICK FRACTURE: *The bone is cracked on one side, bent slightly on both. Such breaks usually affect children, whose bones—like sapling branches—have not fully hardened.*

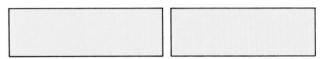

TRANSVERSE FRACTURE: *The bone splits straight across and completely. The lower leg is a frequent site of such fractures; skiing accidents are a common cause.*

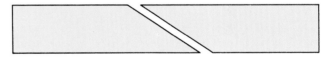

OBLIQUE FRACTURE: *In this break the bone splits completely, as in a transverse fracture, but diagonally. It occurs when the fracturing force is uneven—greater at one end of the bone.*

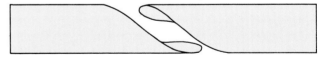

SPIRAL FRACTURE: *Diagonal like the oblique, a spiral fracture also twists the bone, leaving two jagged ends. Such breaks tend to occur in sports that require quick, twisting motions.*

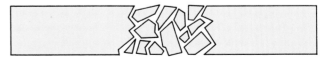

COMMINUTED FRACTURE: *The bone is shattered—broken into three or more pieces. Such breaks usually result from sudden, very violent impacts, such as that occurring after a long fall.*

Crazy Sally, queen of the bonesetters

In 18th Century England, physicians did not bother with the mending of broken bones or dislocated joints. That was the province of an insular and colorful group of practitioners known as bonesetters. Perhaps the most notorious of these was Mrs. Sarah Mapp, better known as Crazy Sally. She learned her craft from her father, a bonesetter in the county of Wiltshire. In the 1730s she hung her shingle in the city of Epsom, winning notice for a formidable physique and a personality to match—both applied with great effect to bonesetting. Reputedly, she reset a dislocated shoulder with the force of her own hands—no mean feat—and straightened a man's leg that had for 20 years been crooked and six inches shorter than his other. "The Lame came to her daily," reported a journal in London, where she eventually set up shop, "and she got a great deal of Money."

Yet to the esteemed British surgeon Percival Pott, Mrs. Mapp was "an ignorant, illiberal, drunken, female savage." Intemperance finally got the better of her, and the renowned Crazy Sally sank into poverty and died at an early age in a London hovel.

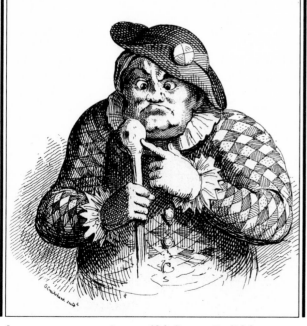

In a contemporary caricature, 18th Century English bonesetter Sarah Mapp—wearing a scowl and the belled cap and motley of a harlequin—examines a distorted human bone, the cartoonist's version of a jester's scepter. Despite this unflattering view, one versifier extolled Mrs. Mapp as "thou wonder of the age," and she counted among her patients many of London's gentry.

lost, creating a shortage even if enough calcium has been consumed in the day's meals.

However, genetic differences in body structure may have more impact than diet on the risk of osteoporosis. People of Oriental descent, who have less total bone mass—smaller and lighter bones—than others, have the greatest incidence of osteoporosis. The risk is highest among Oriental women, who are generally lighter than men. By contrast, black men have the densest bones and suffer the least osteoporosis. Caucasians are in between.

A shortage of vitamin D may also play a part in this bone-thinning process. The so-called sunshine vitamin, supplied by eggs, seafood and fortified milk and activated by the ultraviolet rays of sunlight, stimulates the absorption of calcium and phosphorus through the walls of the intestines. Anyone who does not eat enough of such foods or get enough sunlight suffers because the calcium he consumes stays in the digestive system and never reaches the bones.

Once the damage of osteoporosis has been done, there is no reversing the process. But it is possible to detect the disease early by X-raying the hip to examine the condition of the top section of the thighbone—a naturally honeycombed region where loss in bone mass is readily apparent. Some experts recommend that anyone over the age of 50 should have such an examination and, if it reveals signs of bone loss, should supplement his diet with calcium and vitamin D.

Such a regimen will not replace bone mineral that has been lost; at best, diet supplements may slow the progress of osteoporosis. But the ailment can be prevented: Exercise, moderate weight and a diet that is limited in phosphorus-laden foods but rich in calcium and vitamin D maintain the solidity of the skeleton.

However, those osteoporosis sufferers who also have high blood pressure or heart disease and therefore must limit their cholesterol intake should choose carefully in increasing their intake of calcium and vitamin D. Instead of eggs, whole milk and fatty cheeses, they should use low-fat milk and cottage cheese and also eat plenty of leafy green vegetables.

Healthy bones are not only more resistant to fracture, but are also likely to heal more readily if a break occurs. Healing is accomplished by the same biological processes that steadily build and replenish bone over the course of a lifetime, but the processes accelerate to repair a fracture. Any bone's natural tendency is to repair itself; however, even the strongest bones generally need some mechanical assistance if they are to knit neatly back into their original shape.

Itinerant bonesetter to orthopedic surgeon

From the earliest times, humans have sought ways to help nature perform its restorative bone-building. More than 5,000 years ago physicians in India, China and Egypt were skillfully treating fractures and dislocations. Around the Sixth Century B.C. one Indian medical text devoted an entire chapter to the subject, classifying types of fractures and advising methods to treat each. The ancient Greeks recognized the need for conditioning exercises to keep the muscles of a broken limb from wasting while the bone healed, and they tailored their splints and casts—bandages stiffened with wax and starch—to specific injuries.

With the fall of the ancient world many of these medical skills were lost. In Europe during the Middle Ages, surgery and the orthopedic arts in particular suffered a decline; both were held in low regard, the province of artisans rather than educated physicians. Even into the 19th Century in Britain, surgeons were trained differently from other medical practitioners and were considered inferior to them. Fractures were handled by itinerants known as bonesetters, who passed their skills along from father to son—or daughter: One of the most famous of the 18th Century bonesetters was a woman called Crazy Sally Mapp.

In the 19th Century, many of the ancient techniques were rediscovered, as physicians began to learn how bones heal. British physician Hugh Owen Thomas, descendant of a long line of Welsh bonesetters, in the course of treating injured Liverpool dockworkers developed some of the common fracture splints that are still in use today. Another of his contributions was the discovery that a flow of blood to the site of a fracture was essential to healing. However, his method of spurring the healing flow was crude: He rapped the injured area with a mallet. One of Thomas' patients became so enraged by the painful tapping that he grabbed the mallet and tried—unsuccessfully—to bash in Thomas' head.

The science of bone repair took its greatest strides at the close of the century, with three of medicine's most revolutionary advances. The first was the development of anesthesia; now patients like those of Hugh Thomas could be treated painlessly. The second was antiseptic operating rooms, which lessened the threat of infection and enabled doctors to repair complicated breaks surgically.

The third contribution, and the one most pertinent to orthopedics, came in 1895 when German physicist Wilhelm Conrad Roentgen discovered X-rays. Doctors all over the world were soon familiar with the ghostly outlines of Roentgen's wife's hand bones—the world's first X-ray picture—and were busily devising ways to use the strange phenomenon in their own practices. For those surgeons and for generations since, Roentgen's X-rays provided a view not only of healthy bones but of broken ones as well, enabling doctors to see the nature of virtually any fracture and decide how best to treat it.

Assessing the damage

Today an orthopedist will order X-rays as a matter of course if he suspects a bone is broken. In addition, he will quiz the patient to learn exactly how the accident took place, because such details may point to other injuries or complications—perhaps internal harm or nerve damage.

Sometimes, even given the doctor's questioning and the X-ray's penetrating power, still more information is needed. Perhaps the X-ray shows nothing, yet the patient's pain continues for several days. In most hospitals today the doctor can then order a diagnostic test called a bone scan, which was developed in the late 1950s.

The patient is injected with a drug that has been mixed with a weak radioactive substance, such as technetium 99, which emits gamma rays in tiny doses that pose no threat to human tissues. The drug is a form of phosphorus, and within two to four hours after injection it will adhere to the bone that is starting to bridge the break just as if it were phosphorus from food—taking the ray-emitting technetium along with it.

Much the way a geiger counter is used in prospecting for

Mandavu lies anesthetized on a bed of hay, unaware of the delicate medical work being done by Dr. David Gershuni, who bends over her fractured hind leg, probing for healthy bone. If Mandavu's fracture had not been successfully treated, she would have been put out of her misery.

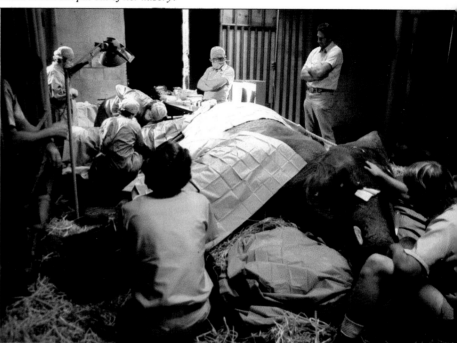

A cast strong enough for an elephant

When an elephant breaks a leg, the problem of restoring health is as big as the patient. Saving a 7,000-pound African female named Mandavu, who fell into an eight-foot moat at San Diego Wild Animal Park and broke her right rear leg, required a 20-man orthopedic team as well as techniques and materials new to the treatment of big animals. Among the revolutionary materials was an ultrastrong plastic used for the cast (it is employed also to set human fractures). Previous efforts to mend big animal bones had involved the use of metal plates, an approach that produced few—and then only partial—successes.

Mandavu could be anesthetized for only about four hours before her lungs would collapse under her weight. After knocking her out with an anesthetic, the team braced the injured leg with eight railroad ties. Next, team leader Dr. David Gershuni made an incision below the knee and drilled a hole through healthy bone above the fracture. He then drove an 18-inch steel pin through the hole, anchoring it to rigid external metal braces on either side of Mandavu's leg. Together the pin and braces immobilized the fractured bone.

Technicians then covered the brace with the cast made from thin polyurethane plastic strips. The strips first were dipped in water, a step that softens them and makes them easier to apply. In seven minutes the cast set firm, yet remained flexible. The finished cast was less than an inch thick and weighed barely three and a half pounds.

After three hours and 22 minutes, the team held its breath while Mandavu was awakened with an antidote to the anesthetic. Struggling to her feet, she put all her weight on the new cast. It held, and her recovery had begun.

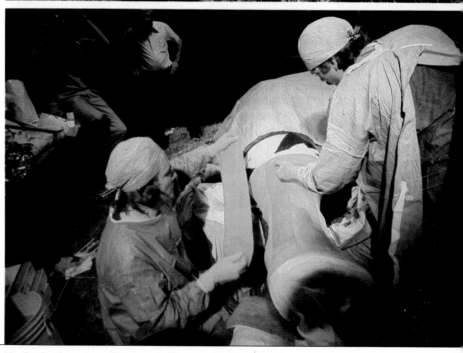

Her broken bones set, Mandavu has her mending leg placed in a special cast. Here casting technicians, who have sheathed the leg in cushioning cotton and polyester stockings, apply layers of polyurethane strips, selected for the task because they are strong enough to bear the elephant's weight yet flexible enough so they will give without cracking.

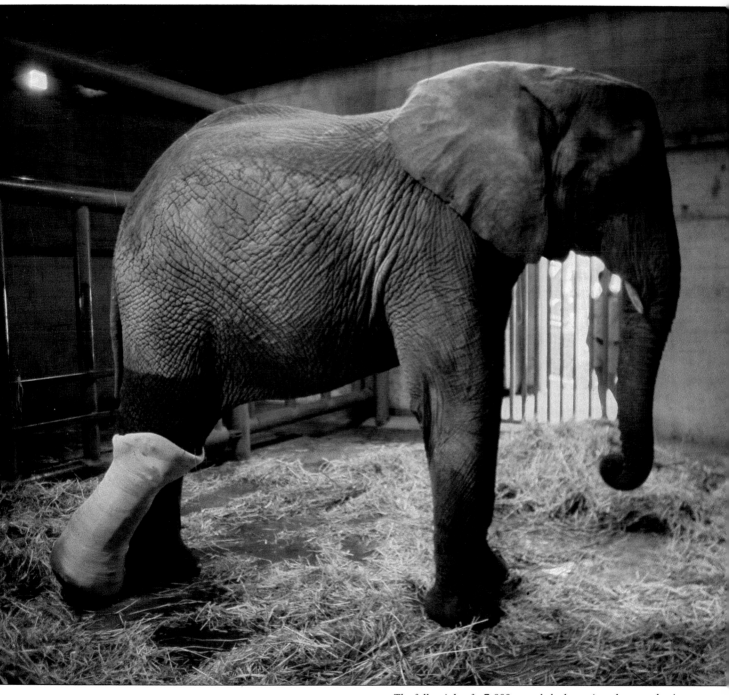

The full weight of a 7,000-pound elephant gives the new plastic cast the ultimate test. According to Dr. Gershuni, Mandavu somehow sensed that it was in her best interest to take it easy on the cast, and not bang it up or tug it off. But because it became grubby and loose, and because doctors needed to check Mandavu's progress, the cast had to be replaced three times.

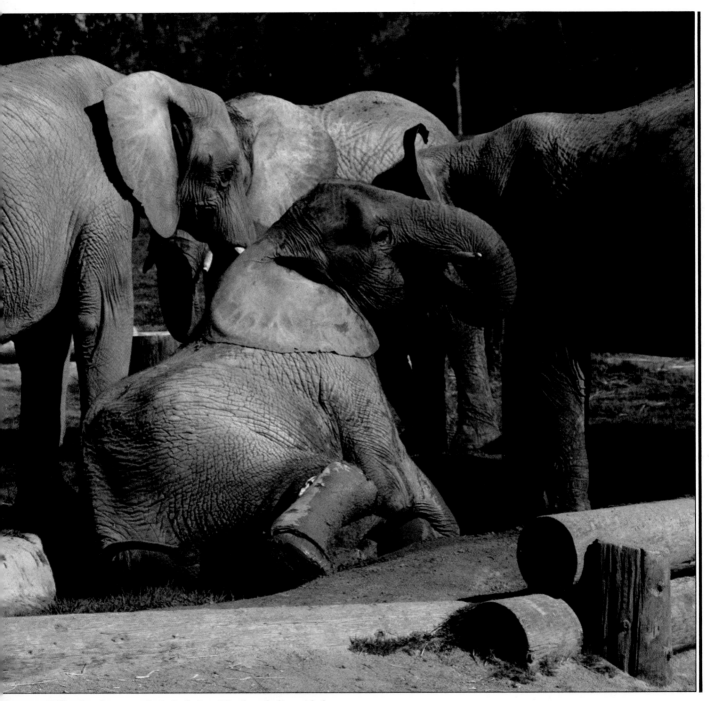

*Following three months in isolation, Mandavu frolics with the
rest of the herd as if the cast were not there. Her playmates,
however, were acutely aware of it. After they deviled the cast
for days, it had to be removed once and for all—but Mandavu's
bones had already healed. Full recovery took a year.*

uranium ores, a detecting device is then moved over the patient (or sometimes the patient is moved under the instrument). Radiation from the bones strikes crystals in the detector, generating a signal that is converted electronically into an image on a television-like screen or recorded on film. What the doctor sees then is not mere anatomy—such as that visible in an X-ray photograph—but the restorative processes in action. As blood flows to the fracture site, the bone, kicking up its activity to mend itself, takes in more nutrients—including the phosphorus carrying its tags of radioactive technetium. The fracture, where this increased activity is going on, shows up as a "hot spot," a more intensely radioactive area than the area surrounding it.

Bone scans are particularly helpful when patients have sustained tiny cracks in the lower leg. "Young military recruits put through lots of running and marching develop those injuries," explained Dr. Harold Goldstein, of the University of Pennsylvania. "Sometimes those recruits aren't trying to slough off; they have pain. This test can distinguish the sloughers from the ones with real injuries."

Once diagnosed, these and other small fractures may need little beyond bandaging to minimize movement. A cracked rib, for example, will heal itself unassisted. The patient is merely advised to rest for a few days. Usually, though, a broken bone must be "reduced"—that is, it must be set.

The fine art of reducing a fracture

Reducing is an art, and orthopedists pride themselves on their touch. How the surgeon proceeds may depend as much on his personal quirks and his estimate of the patient's personality as on the severity of the injury. In most cases, he will first administer an anesthetic, which not only relieves pain but relaxes muscles whose contractions might interfere with manipulation of the bone. Some doctors, however, prefer to work without painkillers whenever humanely possible. A suburban New York housewife who broke her wrist was treated swiftly by an orthopedist who told her, "I have to see how you react to tell how I'm doing." He tugged at the bones, and suddenly her pain stopped—a sure indication that the fragmented bones were in their correct positions.

If the fracture is a simple one, the doctor—sometimes with the aid of an assistant—will pull at the sections of bone to separate them. Then, using gentle but persistent pulling and pushing motions, he will shift the bone segments back together, making sure that the fragments are correctly aligned—neither rotated so as to cause a twisted bone, nor angled to produce a bent one.

Surprisingly, actual abutment of the broken ends is not important, for the doctor knows that the hard-working human body will take care of linking up the sundered parts on its own. In fact, with a very young child, the broken ends may be purposely overlapped an inch or so, for the child's natural growth may be outpaced by the bone-building that repairs a fracture; without the overlapping, an injured bone can end up much longer than its mate.

Aligning bones correctly is a matter of experience, touch and instinct—usually aided by additional X-rays. More than one person suffering from a broken limb has had to climb back on the X-ray table after his arm or leg was set, climb down again so the doctor could make a slight adjustment and then climb back on for another look before the doctor declared his handiwork acceptable. "That," said Dr. James Dickson, a Rye, New York, orthopedist who has done hundreds of reductions, "is the tricky part. You have to be tough on yourself and not hesitate to fix it if it isn't right."

Once the bone has been set, the surgeon will in most cases apply a plaster cast—a means of immobilizing broken bones first used by the Arabs, who poured the wet substance directly over broken limbs perhaps as early as the 16th Century. European bonesetters relied on splints until Antonius Mathijsen, a Dutch army surgeon, devised in 1852 the technique that is still used today.

First the injured area is wrapped in sheet cotton. Then strips of plaster-soaked gauze are laid around it and allowed to dry until firm. The procedure sounds simple, but applying a cast properly is almost as exacting an art as reducing a bone. "When I was an intern," recalled Dr. Dickson, "I always wanted to apply casts but was never allowed to. I couldn't understand why not. Then the day came when I was permitted to do it—and I found out how hard it is."

Trickiest to handle is the cotton sheeting, which must protect the patient's skin from the surprising heat generated by drying plaster; this heat can cause a burn. The cast then must be tight enough to keep joined bone fragments from budging, but not so tight as to impede circulation.

Doctors rarely delegate to assistants the application of the initial cast. If it is done improperly, the doctor learns of the error soon enough. "A few phone calls at 3 a.m. from patients who say their cast hurts terribly and would you please fix it immediately will bring you right back into line," Dr. Dickson observed. If additional casts are needed later, the task may go to a technician because healing has already begun and precise fitting is not essential.

Annoying, inconvenient and cumbersome a cast may be, but it is the price that must be paid for adequate healing. Most patients hate casts, and dread the itching they inevitably cause. Although it sets as hard as a rock, a cast does permit easy adjustments if swelling increases. A doctor can slice the cast lengthwise, separate the two halves slightly and tape them together in that position. The procedure is known as bivalving and is done with a special electric handsaw that can tear through the tough material swiftly without scratching the flesh beneath. It has a rotary blade but the blade does not spin; it turns backward and forward very quickly over a very short distance. The back-and-forth sawing will cut through a stiff material such as plaster; on a soft substance such as flesh, it causes a minor vibration but no damage.

In many cases, plaster can be exchanged after a few weeks for light, water-resistant fiberglass, which "breathes," virtually eliminating itching beneath it. Strips of fiberglass tape impregnated with epoxy resin—much like the patching material used to repair dents in automobiles—are applied in the same way as the original plaster. Another newly developed material may turn out to be better still: resin-coated cotton, lighter even than fiberglass and equally tough.

New ways to aid the worst cases

For some fractures a cast is inadequate. A patient with a broken pelvis may have to repose for six to eight weeks in an orthopedic bed, his lower body encased in a girdle connected to weights that exert a gentle, steady pull. One with a broken leg may be similarly outfitted, but with weights attached to his body by metal pins that are inserted through the skin and driven into uninjured bones near the site of the fracture.

Occasionally a break will be so bad—the bones smashed into several fragments or perhaps the ends jammed into each other—that yet another method must be used, both to maneuver the bones into position and to fix them in place. In many such cases, a surgeon can use a technique called external fixation. Through small incisions, he drills tiny holes into each bone fragment, then inserts wires or pins into the holes. These are fastened to a metal frame outside the body. The doctor uses the wires like puppet strings, to guide the fragments into place; he then tightens the nuts that hold the wires or pins to the external frame. The entire apparatus functions like a cast and is left in place until the break heals.

If the fracture is too complex to be reduced by manipulation from without, or if the bone has broken through the skin, the doctor must perform open surgery. He bares the bones, maneuvers the various parts or fragments together and anchors them with screws, rods or plates. Doctors refer to this method as internal fixation. The hardware, exquisitely crafted of materials such as stainless steel, Teflon, polyethylene and a cobalt-chromium alloy called vitallium, generally is surgically removed after the bone has healed. In some cases—if the damage was extensive or if an elderly patient has very brittle bones—the devices stay inside the body, as permanent reinforcement for the weakened skeleton.

No matter how broken bones are brought back together, they always mend themselves in the same way, starting the moment the fracture occurs. Blood gathers around the break, forming a sticky mass that within hours becomes a thick blood clot. The clot fills the space between and around the bone ends—which in most cases have already been brought together by the doctor—and serves as the basis for what will be new bone. Within a day the jelly-like clot has undergone a further change: It has been invaded by the two kinds of cells needed for healing, osteoclasts and osteoblasts. Osteoclasts, which break down bone and ready it for renewal, dissolve the jagged edges of the old, broken bone. At the same time, osteoblasts—which create new bone—begin to build a network of cells in the clot. Soon the clot takes on a granular quality and begins to seem like a bridge linking the bones.

As the osteoblast network continues to build, the clot is slowly absorbed by the body and the bridge turns into a chalklike callus. Loosely holding the bone pieces together, the callus is at first not very strong—any abrupt motion can tear the union apart—but in time, the body deposits calcium in the callus, further hardening it and eventually converting it into solid bone. Soon it is strong enough to bear weight.

When the bridge is first formed, it is usually larger than the bone it is joining, so that on an X-ray it appears as an olive-shaped bulge around the fracture. For many months it retains its bulgy contour. Then, as the bone hardens further under increasing use, the osteoclasts eat away the extra material, and in a year or two the new bone is indistinguishable from the rest of the body's bony structure. In many cases it is actually stronger than the bone it has supplanted and, particularly in a young person, no sign of the fracture will remain. It is almost as if nothing had ever happened at all.

Sometimes, though, even bones that have been set perfectly will not heal. Because of an infection, an obstruction to the blood supply or some congenital malfunction of the system, the natural process does not work. The bone manufactures soft tissue to link the sundered parts, but the body cannot take the next step: transforming the soft tissue into new bone. The unfortunate victim of this nonunion, as physicians call fractures that do not heal, may be left permanently disabled. In recent years, however, doctors and scientists have discovered that when bones so damaged are stimulated by currents of electricity, in many cases they will knit together.

In 1976 New York insurance broker Julie Wiener fractured his leg in a bizarre auto accident. He had been trying to close the car door when the vehicle started to roll and, as he told magazine writer Lally Weymouth, ''I ran over myself with my own car.'' His leg was properly treated, but after two and a half years in a cast, it had not healed and amputation seemed likely. In a last-ditch attempt to save the leg, Wiener spent 20 months immobile while his limb was bombarded with electrical currents. Finally he set a deadline—May 12, 1980: After that, he would have the leg removed. That drastic move was never necessary. Two days after the deadline, Julie Wiener went shopping and bought ''something I thought I'd never wear again—a pair of shoes.''

The process that put Wiener back on his feet is based on the so-called piezoelectric effect. This is a phenomenon that affects all kinds of solid substances, including bone: Solid objects, when subjected to an electrical force, develop a mechanical stress. Stress makes bone grow—that is why exercise strengthens bone. Thus the application of a stress-

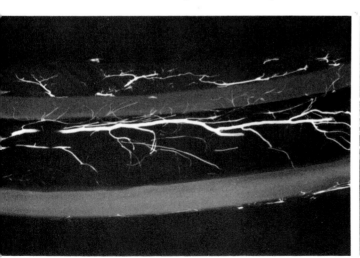

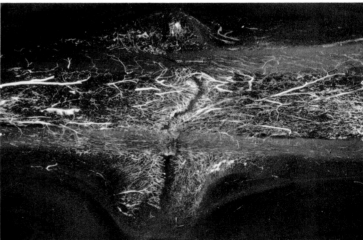

How a dog's broken bone heals is shown by these special X-rays contrasting a healthy leg (above, left) with one fractured six weeks earlier. Human fractures heal the same way. The blood vessels, injected with dye that makes them stand out in X-rays, are visible as large, branching arteries in healthy bone, but primarily as a jumble of tiny capillaries in the slowly healing bone. The capillaries nourish specialized cells that dissolve jagged edges of dead bone at the central break; they also sustain another variety of cell that builds new bone in the large bulges of callus at the edges of the break. When the bone is fully healed, the callus almost completely disappears and normal blood vessels bridge the fracture.

inducing electrical force to bone apparently induces the growth of tissue. New bone cells grow to bridge the gap in a fracture and the break heals.

Electricity may be applied to the bone in three ways. The method used on Julie Wiener's leg was devised by Dr. Andrew Bassett and his colleagues at Columbia University. Magnetic coils are placed on either side of the fracture area for as many as 12 hours each day. The coils set up electrical forces that spur cell activity within the limb. Another device, developed by Drs. Carl T. Brighton and Z. B. Friedenberg of the University of Pennsylvania, delivers current more directly, through electrodes planted under the patient's skin; power is supplied by a battery implanted in the cast. Even more self-contained is a mechanism that is totally implanted, power pack and all, within the body.

For the patient, there are trade-offs, especially with the first and the last of these methods. With Dr. Bassett's coils, a patient takes no surgical risks but he must stay in one place, hooked up to the force-producing box, for long periods. With the total implant, the patient is free to move about while the electrical stimulation is going on, but he also has to undergo the operation that puts the unit into his body and may suffer postoperative complications. Such drawbacks aside, however, all three methods work.

Electrical stimulation is an experimental and highly speculative technique that has aroused considerable controversy. Some experts think it could cause cancer. The artificial acceleration of cell growth might cause the production of abnormal cells. One of the pioneers in electrical stimulation, Dr. Robert Becker of Upstate Medical Center of the State University of New York, cautioned against the routine use of the method for speeding normal healing. "The process of healing is based on cell multiplication and increased activity. The malignant process is not far removed from the normal healing process, so before there's any clinical use of electrical stimulation to make a normal healing process go faster, I believe it is absolutely essential that basic research be done to evaluate the safety of that technique," he said. "You don't accept the risk of starting a malignant process just to give the patient two weeks back on the job."

For a little girl who had been about to lose her leg after enduring 10 operations for a shinbone that would not heal, such conservative caution was not applicable. Taking her last chance for a life with two normal limbs, she became Dr. Bassett's first electrical-stimulation patient in 1973. "In four months," he recalled, "she healed, and that was the end of her problem. It was the first time that she had ever been healed in her eight years of life."

Putting Humpty Dumpty together with man-made bone

Some fractures cannot be set in a way that would allow any bone-repairing process, either spontaneous or stimulated. Such bones, like Humpty Dumpty, are so badly damaged they they cannot be put back together again. For them, a substitute must be found.

In the case of a crushed joint—where not only bone but also cartilage has been destroyed—an artificial replacement of metal and plastic can be installed. First the damaged area is removed entirely. Then the replacement, or prosthesis, which has been trimmed at both ends to fit the space, is cemented to the remaining bone. Although such spare parts are used most often to replace joints ravaged by arthritis, they also make excellent substitutes for fractured hips, shoulders and elbows.

In some cases where a fracture has left a wide gap in a bone, the body can be induced to manufacture its own replacement part. The most common method of doing this involves the bone graft. A piece of bone is taken from another part of the patient's body and used to bridge the gap. The graft is not a permanent replacement part in itself: It is a living scaffold. Eventually, like any other living bone, it will gradually wear out and be absorbed into the body. But in the meantime it will be tolerated by the body; new cells will appear, knitting themselves to the fragments that the graft links and building a strong new unit.

Bone grafts can work seeming miracles. A 28-year-old woman, her right tibia—the larger bone of the lower leg—pulverized by a car crash, was fitted with a long sliver taken from her left fibula, the smaller leg bone. Her body built up new bone in both legs: New cells covered and eventually

Using electricity to heal the unhealable

Five per cent of fractures refuse to heal on their own, for reasons that often cannot be found. Until the early 1970s the only remedies were complicated bone reconstruction, surgery or amputation. Then experiments undertaken by a number of institutions demonstrated that electricity, when applied directly to such stubborn fractures, or nonunions, could make them heal.

In one method, pioneered at the University of Pennsylvania by Dr. Carl Brighton *(right),* four wires, each barely $1/20$ inch thick, are implanted in the bone near the fracture. These wires then are hooked up to a battery, and the whole assembly is covered with a light cast. For 12 weeks the battery continuously sends a tiny current—only about $1/100,000$ the amount that is necessary to light a 100-watt bulb—to the break, stimulating bone growth there.

How electricity helps bones heal is only partly understood. Apparently it induces a mechanical stress in bone cells, and stress makes the special bone-building cells called osteoblasts work harder. Though the process itself remains somewhat mysterious, the results are plain: Nearly 85 per cent of the nonunions heal completely.

Bone expert Dr. Carl Brighton studies four X-rays of his work on leg fractures that failed to heal. Visible in each are the fine wires he inserted to carry electricity to the break and stimulate its repair. In the X-ray second from the bottom, Dr. Brighton can discern the square shape of the battery that supplies the current, and the oval form of a positive electrode, or anode, that is stuck onto the skin.

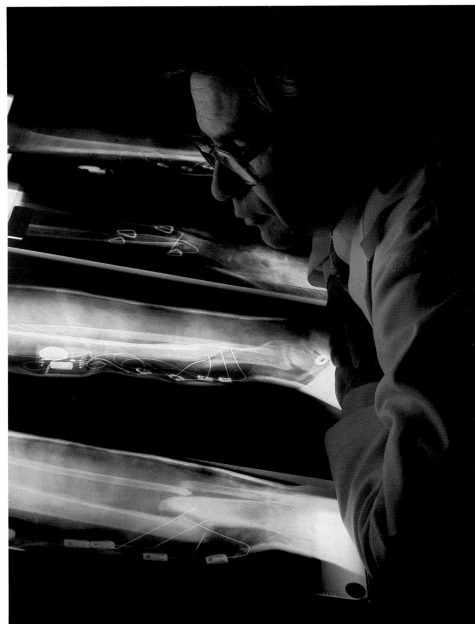

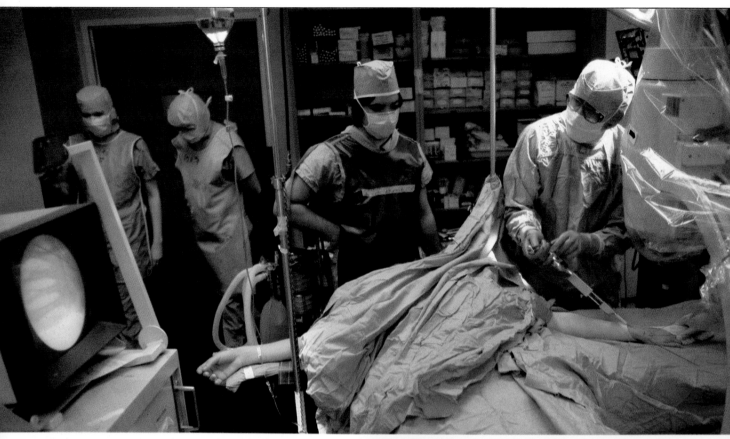

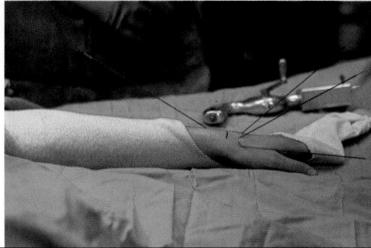

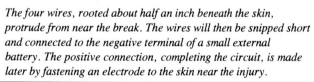

Watching a monitor that televises an X-ray close-up of his work, Dr. Brighton drills a fine hole to insert a stainless-steel wire into the break in a patient's wrist. The electricity the wires carry to promote healing is too faint for the patient to feel.

The four wires, rooted about half an inch beneath the skin, protrude from near the break. The wires will then be snipped short and connected to the negative terminal of a small external battery. The positive connection, completing the circuit, is made later by fastening an electrode to the skin near the injury.

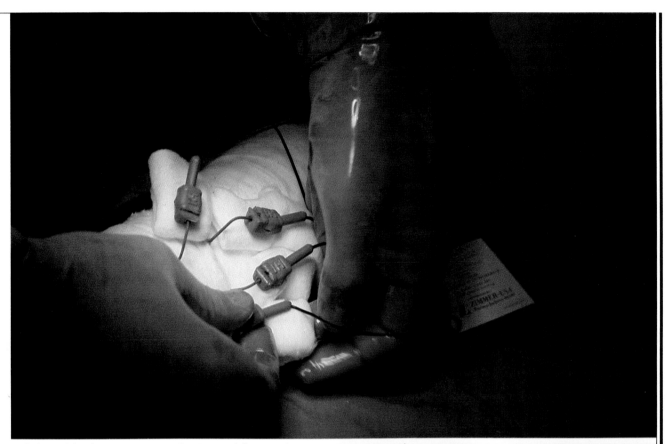

With the pad for the positive connection (upper right corner)
ready to be attached to the arm, Dr. Brighton clamps the last of
the wires protruding from the broken bone, to complete the
negative connection and start the healing current flowing.

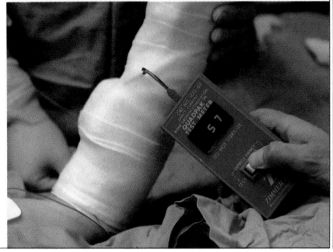

Attached to a monitoring lead emerging from the finished
bandages, a meter reveals that the battery, snug under its covering
of gauze, is still building the current to its normal level of 80
microamperes. In about 12 weeks the wires can be pulled out, but
the bone will require another 12 weeks before it is fully healed.

supplanted the graft in her right one to create a sturdy new tibia, while the same process replaced the bone that had been carved from her left limb. In time, she had the full use of both legs with only a few scars to show for her trouble.

Many other patients, particularly those whose injuries are extensive, cannot spare enough bone to supply what is needed. A piece taken from a live human donor, or still-living bone taken from a just-deceased one, is not the answer. A transplant of this kind is likely to be rejected the way transplanted organs such as kidneys and hearts often are, because such bone, like other foreign tissue introduced into the body, triggers immunological responses.

Dead bones, however, do not cause such a rejection reaction. So bones that have been taken from cadavers and preserved by freezing are used instead. These do not function in the same fashion as bone grafts from the patient's own body. The frozen transplants are dead, so they cannot manufacture new cells of their own and cannot knit themselves to the living bone. They are simply mechanical parts, which are fixed into place with metal plates and cement, just as if they were artificial prostheses.

However, such implants have the ability to inspire biological activity, even if they are incapable of it themselves. The dead bone apparently delivers a ''cell-growth factor''— which may be an electrical charge or the release of some chemical—that stimulates the nearby live bone to manufacture extra new cells. These cells then form a cluster around the union between the dead and the live bone, providing vital support for the connection.

In a variation on this technique, bones from cadavers are crushed and then soaked in hydrochloric acid to remove all of the minerals. The fragments—cut into strips or chips, or ground into powder—are dried, sterilized and stored. When mixed with a saline solution, and worked into an oatmeal-like paste, the powdered bone can be used as a kind of surgical caulk to fill in holes, cracks or other irregularities in living bone. Larger fragments can be used to bridge large gaps.

Like frozen bones used as transplants, the demineralized material stimulates the growth of new bone cells—but in a different manner. Instead of inspiring the bones that it touches to step up their bone-producing activity, it affects the body's fibroblasts, the cells that work to produce scar tissue. When fibroblasts make contact with the implanted material, explained biochemist Julie Glowacki, of Boston's Children's Hospital, ''they change their personality. They change their behavior and become skeletal-producing cells.'' No one knows just why scar-producing fibroblasts turn into bone-building osteoblasts, but the conversion may be affected by an electrical signal from demineralized bone.

In one particularly dramatic application combining several of these techniques, surgeons at the hospital deliberately broke a six-year-old boy's congenitally misshapen, three-lobed skull and removed the bones, temporarily leaving his brain protected only by its covering of tough, fibrous membrane. They crushed the bones into penny-sized chips and demineralized them in acid. Then, using two fresh rib grafts from the boy's own chest for scaffolding, the surgeons recovered the fibrous membrane enveloping his brain with these now-rubbery chips and frosted them over with bone paste. In three months, X-rays revealed signs of bone hardening; in a year, the child had a brand-new skull.

For rapid recovery, keep active

Most fracture victims never need bone grafts, implants or electrical stimulation. If a broken bone has been set properly and nothing has occurred to disturb the union, the patient can come out of the cast on schedule. Long before the cast is removed, the doctor will have started the patient on a rehabilitation program—by urging him to lead an active life. The peril of all bone injuries is that the prolonged immobilization required for healing may cause the muscles to atrophy. So doctors recommend as much general activity as possible, to exercise the muscles—and to keep blood pumping to the fracture area. The stepladder victim with the broken wrists found that even with a cast on each arm he could drive his car, obtain research materials from the library and operate his typewriter—and his surgeon applauded.

Yet even a fracture victim who stays active is chagrined to discover, when freed of his cast, that the mended limb, which felt so secure in its cast, turns out to be woefully thin and discolored, extraordinarily weak and also unaccountably stiff. Only then does he realize that immobility takes its toll, and that a fracture involves a great deal more than the mere breaking of a bone.

As one surgeon described it, "A fracture can be characterized as damage to soft tissue—complicated by a broken bone." When the body receives a blow severe enough to break a bone, muscles are likely to tear, blood vessels to rupture and other connecting tissues to give way. Ironically, the bone itself is the first to mend completely; the rest follows. But the soft tissue's healing processes are wonderfully effective, too. Even blood vessels that have been totally severed will miraculously find their way back together—they send out tiny cellular feelers that eventually hook up, and the blood can flow again.

To speed these mending processes and ensure their success, most doctors specify a rigorous program to bring those enfeebled bones, muscles and joints back into shape. First, to enhance circulation, the limb is bathed and moved about in warm water, a process repeated several times a day for about two weeks until normal color and appearance are regained. Strength returns through exercises tailored to the injured member; most involve working with weights.

The key exercises, however, are aimed at restoring mobility. Only a fracture victim can truly appreciate how easily and how far ordinary mortals can bend. Joints emerging from a cast barely seem to move. Yet they must be pushed, bent, stretched—anything to get them going again. Anyone rehabilitating a broken wrist, for instance, must exercise the joint to free up three separate motions: moving the hand up and down, moving it from side to side, and twisting it from palms-up to palms-down and back. The exercises can be painful—especially the twisting one, which involves holding a hammer by its handle and rotating it. Once used to the hammer, the patient on the mend graduates to a baseball bat.

Gradually it all comes back. Residual swelling finally disappears. The arm or leg looks and feels normal again. For several years the victim may be able to sense an imminent rainstorm from a twinge of pain in the fracture area, because so many extra vessels grew to supply nourishing fluids to the healing injury. When barometric pressure drops, this dense bed of vessels expands—the internal pressure of its fluids remains the same, but air pressure on the body decreases, so that the fluid pressure pushes the vessel walls outward—and this expansion inside the body hurts. Eventually this and all other signs of the fracture will probably depart.

Yet there will be a permanent change, perhaps very subtle. Either consciously or unconsciously the newly repaired person will be just a trifle more careful. The feeling was expressed by a man who fractured a foot bone while carrying a box to his basement. "Now I am less reckless," he said, "I look where I am going. I think about slipping when I am running. I jump less. When I skip the bottom two rungs on a ladder to get to the ground quicker, I think about landing on two feet, with equal weight on both. It's a caution I'm not used to, one that infuriates me, but I am committed to avoiding another injury."

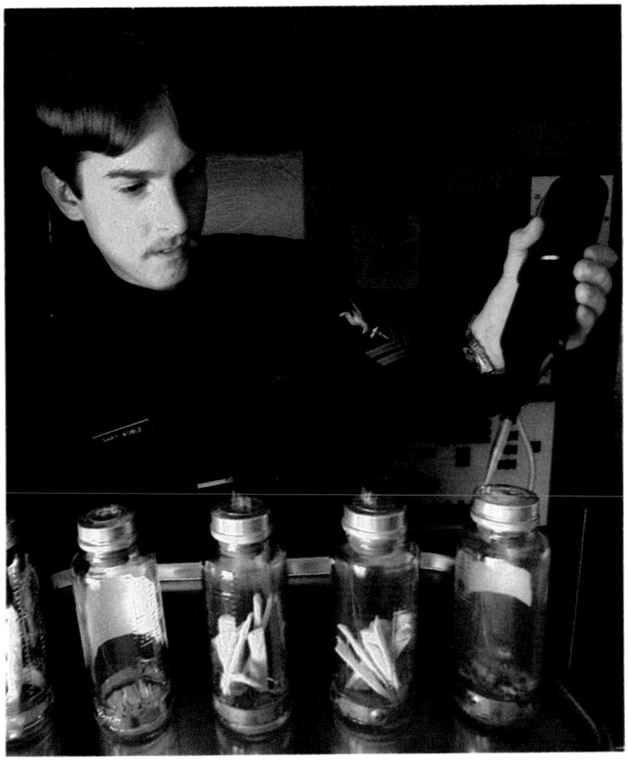

A Navy hospital corpsman uses a device called a spark-tester to check the sterility of human bone taken from cadavers and destined to replace badly shattered bone in fracture victims. The tool generates static electricity on the container: If the container glows with a bluish light, a vacuum has been maintained, assuring sterility, and the bone is ready for transplantation.

CHAPTER 6

Conquering the agony of arthritis

Pinpointing causes and cures
What climate can and cannot do
The diet connection in gout
When quick treatment counts
Making sound choices from an arsenal of drugs
From mystical medicines to copper bracelets
How joints are repaired—or replaced

An executive who had once played professional baseball vividly recalled the day the acute pain of arthritis first assaulted his body's joints. "I was 36 years old, and it was during a softball game in Central Park in New York, and I noticed a little child crawling up the screen behind the batter's cage. I was afraid she'd fall, so I started to go after her, and suddenly I couldn't move my arms from the shoulders. I had to inch myself up the screen by my fingers in order to reach her. That was the first attack; I had a second not long afterward during an evening I spent at home. The second attack was just as unexpected, but much worse—my children had to carry me down the stairs in the morning. Then the attacks came more often and got so bad I wanted to kill myself," he remembered. "So I went to the family physician, who ran some tests and decided I was suffering from gout."

Had he really been afflicted with that peculiar joint ailment, he would have been made better quickly by the special diet and the antigout drug, allopurinol, his doctor prescribed. But the episodic attacks of joint pain recurred, sending him to another doctor and finally to a third who, after more tests, ventured a diagnosis.

" 'I'm pretty sure I know what you have—rheumatoid arthritis. But,' " the executive recalled him cautioning, " 'before you start thinking you're going to end up a cripple, I want to say this: You have two things in your favor: First, you're in good shape, and second, you're a male. In some males, the arthritis is not as acute as in females. But you will have to work with me—and work hard—to keep it under control. If so, you can feel better and lead a near-normal life. Of all my patients,' " he added, " 'there is only one in a wheelchair. And that's because she wants to be. She won't move; she won't help herself.' "

Ten years later this patient had proved his doctor right. Still following a carefully planned program of rest, exercise and a course of medication—in his case, the treatment consisted of injections of compounds containing gold—he was once again leading a full life. "I play tennis, softball. I hurt occasionally; just the other day my wrist hurt, but that was my own fault because I was forcing some golf shots. I manage to travel on business; I once did seven cities in 10 days, although that probably was pushing it. When I travel like that, I carry some powerful tablets—prednisone, a drug that reduces joint inflammation—but luckily I've only had to take one in four years."

His ordeal and its outcome—grappling with excruciating pain, seeking out a doctor familiar with arthritis' puzzling symptoms, reaching the correct diagnosis and coming to grips with the disease—parallel the experiences of most people struck with the outstanding scourge of the body's system of bones and muscles. Arthritis is an ancient crippler; Neanderthal man's celebrated hunched-over stance was caused by it, and evidences of the ailment have been detected in Egyptian mummies. It is not one illness, but many—including the rheumatoid arthritis of the athletic executive, the osteoarthritis of the elderly and that awful pain in the big toe, gout. At least 100 different types of disease that attack the joints are

Taut cords of rubber, laced through a plastic frame, provide therapeutic exercise for a woman whose hand has been stiffened by arthritis. By alternately pushing and pulling on the cords, she limbers the swollen, tight joints of her fingers.

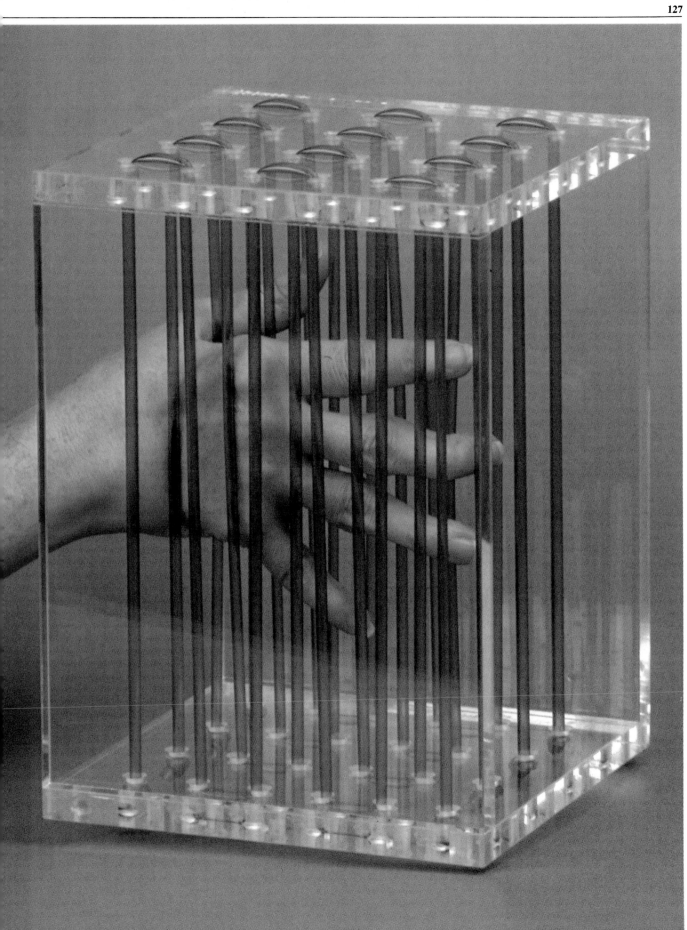

loosely grouped under the heading of arthritis, sometimes called rheumatism. They have in common only their general symptoms: joint pain and loss of motion. They differ in their causes and in the damage they do.

According to one source, this large group of diseases causes more invalidism in Western countries than any other conditions except heart disease and mental illness. It can strike the young—many thousands of children suffer from it—as well as the old. It can come on slowly or it can swoop down upon an unsuspecting victim with punishing swiftness. It may depart suddenly, leaving no symptoms behind—then inexplicably reappear. Its economic impact in the United States alone comes to some $14.5 billion a year in doctors' bills, medications, lost wages and other costs.

For some of the most relentless types of arthritis there is no agreed-upon cause, and no real cure. It is a chronic ailment: Once afflicted, a victim is likely to be permanently susceptible. To many arthritis sufferers its onset and seemingly vindictive course can be so devastating that they often resort in desperation to useless nostrums and dangerously inappropriate cures; Americans waste an estimated $950 million on these frauds each year.

Pinpointing causes and cures

Yet this baffling and complex group of ailments should not evoke despair. Today it can be diagnosed readily in its early, treatable stages, and prompt treatment may prevent its crippling effects. Even its elusive causes are being uncovered. The origins of some types are known. Gout results from a build-up of uric acid, a normal body waste product; several kinds of arthritis result directly from infection. And one factor in rheumatoid arthritis may be the regulatory substances related to gender—three times as many women as men come down with rheumatoid arthritis. Of women sufferers who become pregnant, three out of four experience extraordinary relief; in their hunt for the cause of these remissions, researchers are focusing attention on a substance called pregnancy alpha-glycoprotein, which may be generated in the course of pregnancy by the female sex hormone. Said Dr. Frederic McDuffie, a senior vice president of the Arthritis Foundation, "It's a jigsaw puzzle, and we're down to the last few pieces."

Today the search for those missing pieces is centering on the body's immune system—a breakdown in this defense system seems to set up several forms of arthritis. The agent of such a breakdown may be a virus or bacteria, which could cause the body's defender cells—white blood cells—to turn into attackers that damage joint tissue. If such an agent proves to be the enemy, it might be inactivated and made into a vaccine to prevent arthritis.

Although the causes of all forms of arthritis remain to be established, new and better ways to halt their progress are being found. Experimental radiation treatments and blood-cleansing techniques similar to those used successfully to eliminate excess white blood cells in cancer patients are being tested in an attempt to block the damage such cells apparently cause in arthritis. New drugs such as azathioprine also suppress the immune system, while others such as ibuprofen reduce inflammation quickly. Older medicines are being improved. For example, periodic injections of gold have helped many people since the 1920s, but the shots are painful and can also bring such side effects as kidney damage, skin rash and diarrhea. Recently, different compounds of gold have been developed that can be taken in pill form rather than by injection; this method of preparing the drug permits more frequent administration of smaller doses and may reduce some of the unpleasant side effects.

For the legions of arthritis sufferers who might once have spent their lives hobbling about on canes because a hip or knee joint was damaged, repairs are available. If the original joint has been destroyed, it can be replaced. Metal and plastic substitutes not only restore full movement but can prevent additional damage that might result from a crippled posture. And at the University of Texas Southwestern Medical School, doctors are using new surgical procedures to remove diseased bone and supplant it with healthy bone. The replacement bone has its normal cartilage attached, to provide cushioning for pain-free movement.

Today only a small percentage of all victims are genuinely disabled or even greatly inconvenienced. According to Dr.

Ephraim Engleman of the University of California Medical School, the chance that anyone who contracts even the severest forms of the disease will become totally disabled is now probably no more than 3 out of 100.

Once doctors felt compelled to tell their newly diagnosed arthritis patients, ''I'm sorry, but nothing can be done.'' Now they can echo the words of Dr. John Calabro, who said, ''I have never met an arthritis patient I could not help, no matter how severe or far advanced the arthritis may be.'' Added Dr. Harry Spiera of New York's Mt. Sinai Hospital, ''Most people, when they think of arthritis, visualize a deformed person with gnarled joints huddled in a wheelchair. Little do they realize that all around them, on the streets and in offices and stores, are people who have one or another of the varieties of the disease but who have it under complete and successful control.''

Such an encouraging prognosis can be made for those who recognize the symptoms and get to a doctor early. Delay in diagnosis and treatment may cause unnecessary crippling because the vital joint-cushioning cartilage that makes movement possible cannot be replaced once it has been destroyed, whether by a dramatic attack of the immune system or by nothing more than a lack of exercise. Of the two, a lack of exercise is the more insidious, but it is just as devastating in its effects. Because of pain on movement, the victim simply stops trying to move the joint. Then, without exercise, supporting muscles weaken and shorten, reducing and eventually destroying the range of motion. If medication is promptly initiated, though, it alleviates pain and inflammation. The arthritis sufferer then can begin the important physical therapy—mild exercises alternating with rest for the joints—that will prevent further harm to those remarkable mechanisms that allow human beings to walk, talk, sit, stand, throw a ball, hug a friend and run for the pure joy of it.

A vulnerable marvel of engineering

The typical joint is a wonder of engineering—at least when it is working properly. Each of the two bones making up the joint is faced with a layer of cartilage up to an eighth of an inch thick that acts both to cushion the bones and to enable

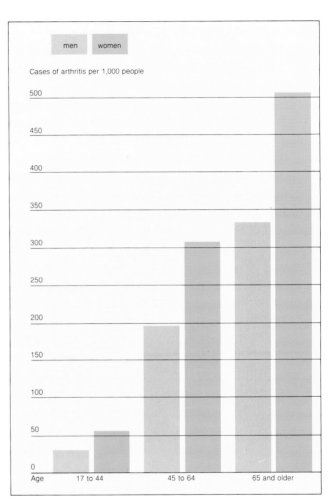

ARTHRITIS: A SPECIAL RISK FOR WOMEN.
For reasons yet unknown, women of all ages face a greater threat of arthritis than men do. More predictably, figures compiled by the National Center for Health Statistics and graphed above demonstrate that arthritis is rare in children and increases with age in both sexes; more than half the women over 65 suffer some form of the disease. Arthritis is even more common than the figures indicate—victims of gout and arthritis-prone residents of nursing homes or other institutions were not counted.

The four types of arthritis

Doctors identify more than 100 different kinds of arthritis, but most fit into one of four categories, each characterized by a pattern of joint deterioration *(right)*—a way in which a healthy joint *(below)* goes awry and afflicts the victim with pain, tenderness, stiffness and restricted movement.

The two most common types, rheumatoid arthritis *(top right)* and osteoarthritis *(bottom right),* make up more than two thirds of all cases. They develop slowly from uncertain causes and usually result in cartilage damage, but the basic similarities end there. In rheumatoid arthritis, the synovial membranes *(red)* become inflamed; in osteoarthritis, the joint becomes disfigured because the bone ends thicken and roughen as if to compensate for the damaged cartilage.

In the two other major categories of arthritis, gout *(second from top)* and infectious arthritis *(second from bottom),* the causes are better understood. Contaminants—either body wastes, such as unprocessed uric-acid crystals, or bacteria—injure the cartilage and impair its cushioning ability.

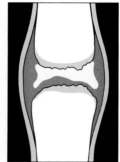

RHEUMATOID ARTHRITIS: INFLAMMATION
Inflamed, swollen synovial membranes (red) are the primary signs of rheumatoid arthritis, the major crippling form of the disease. In such inflammatory arthritis, the membranes produce excess fluid that distends the joint and frequently causes severe pain and stiffness.

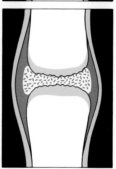

GOUT FROM A FLAW IN BODY CHEMISTRY
In gout and in at least two other forms of crystalline arthritis, inadequately processed waste products (black specks) collect in the synovial fluid, triggering painful inflammation. The villain in gout, the most common form, is uric-acid crystals, which accumulate primarily in the big toe.

INFECTION'S OMINOUS "HOT JOINT"
Staphylococcus, gonococcus and tuberculosis bacteria, well known as threats to the body's organs, can also infect the synovial fluid and produce painful swelling, redness and heat—the so-called hot joint of infectious arthritis.

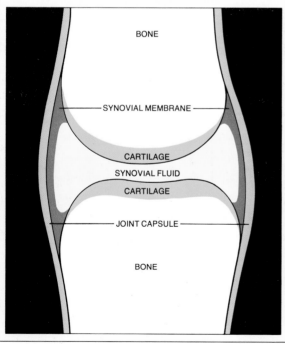

BONE

SYNOVIAL MEMBRANE

CARTILAGE
SYNOVIAL FLUID
CARTILAGE

JOINT CAPSULE

BONE

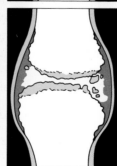

JOINT DEGENERATION: OSTEOARTHRITIS
In osteoarthritis, cartilage thins, cracks and breaks away, often leaving bone ends unprotected. Bone ends roughen and thicken, disfiguring the joint. This is far and away the most prevalent form of arthritis.

NORMAL JOINTS: WELL-OILED MACHINES
A joint is a neatly integrated cushioning system: Inside its fibrous capsule, the synovial membrane exudes a fluid to nourish and lubricate cartilage. Together, cartilage, membrane and fluid absorb shocks and prevent friction.

them to slide easily against each other. Their motion is eased by a liquid known as synovial fluid, so called because it looks like *(syn-)* the white of an egg *(ovum)*. The fluid is secreted by the synovial membrane, a layer of tissue as transparently thin as plastic food wrap. Outside this membrane is another, tougher layer of fibrous tissue called the joint capsule, itself surrounded by tissue punctuated with fluid-filled sacs—the bursae—that are buffers for the friction of the tendons. When one of the elements of a joint wears out or is damaged by disease, the result is arthritis. What happens to which element determines the type of arthritis.

One susceptible element is the layer of cartilage that cushions the bones in a joint. Should it degenerate from excessive stress or perhaps, as one theory suggests, from chemical abnormalities, the joint loses its mobility and the result is osteoarthritis—the wear-and-tear disease that afflicts numberless elderly people.

Other target spots in the joints of some genetically susceptible people are the ligaments in the spine; when they become inflamed, the entire spinal column can freeze up. This form of arthritis has an almost unpronounceable medical name, ankylosing spondylitis, but at its worst it is more commonly and aptly called poker spine. The lubricating synovial fluid is also attacked in gout; the fluid accumulates uric acid in such concentration that the acid solidifies as crystals. And the synovial membrane and bursae are susceptible to infections of many kinds—from streptococcus bacteria to a germ carried by a tick—causing fever and hot, swollen joints.

Inflamed joints are also symptoms of the complex ailment that goes by the name of systemic lupus erythematosus, lupus for short. Lupus is the Latin word for wolf, and a distinguishing feature of the disease can be a red rash that resembles a wolf bite, over the nose and cheeks. The ailment is considered part of the arthritis family because more than three fourths of its victims sooner or later develop joint pain like that of rheumatoid arthritis.

Of all arthritis' many types, by far the most serious as well as the most mystifying is rheumatoid arthritis, characterized by prolonged inflammation of the synovial membrane. This great crippler afflicts six and a half million people in the United States. Capable of generating pain that one patient described as resembling "hot pokers driven into your skin," rheumatoid arthritis strikes in peculiar patterns.

The initial symptoms are likely to be pain and stiffness, followed by tenderness and swelling in symmetrical joints—if several knuckles of the left hand hurt, so do one or more of the right. Why the pain is symmetrical is one of its many mysteries, as is another characteristic: Usually only the middle joints of the fingers are affected, not the ends.

Later the inflammation may spread to other joints or skip around erratically. Muscles and joints are likely to be stiff in the morning, then loosen up during the day. The pain may be accompanied by what might be called misery-all-over symptoms: fatigue, loss of appetite, general weakness and fever. For a victim beset by this combination of symptoms, the simplest daily activities pose obstacles that seem almost insurmountable. One victim recalled that during his worst episode even putting his socks on was painful; he had to use two hands to lift a phone book; walking two blocks to go to work took half an hour. "You don't know what it is," he said, "until you've had the pain of arthritis. It can make you sick to your stomach. Once when I was driving my car I felt pain in my neck that made me so dizzy I had to pull over to the side of the road until it went away."

What brings on the agony of rheumatoid arthritis has been the subject of research, speculation and hot debate for centuries. Some theories, however, have proved to be far more credible than others.

Until the 1940s, some physicians based a common remedy for the disease on the mistaken belief that the bacteria in decaying teeth spread poison through the system; they ordered all the patient's teeth extracted, a drastic and useless procedure. An improper diet has also been blamed, but today doctors are convinced that diet is irrelevant except as it bears on the patient's overall fitness and resistance to disease.

What climate can and cannot do

Similarly baseless is the blame laid on cold and damp climates. If environment were a cause, then more people would be expected to have arthritis in the dank of England than in

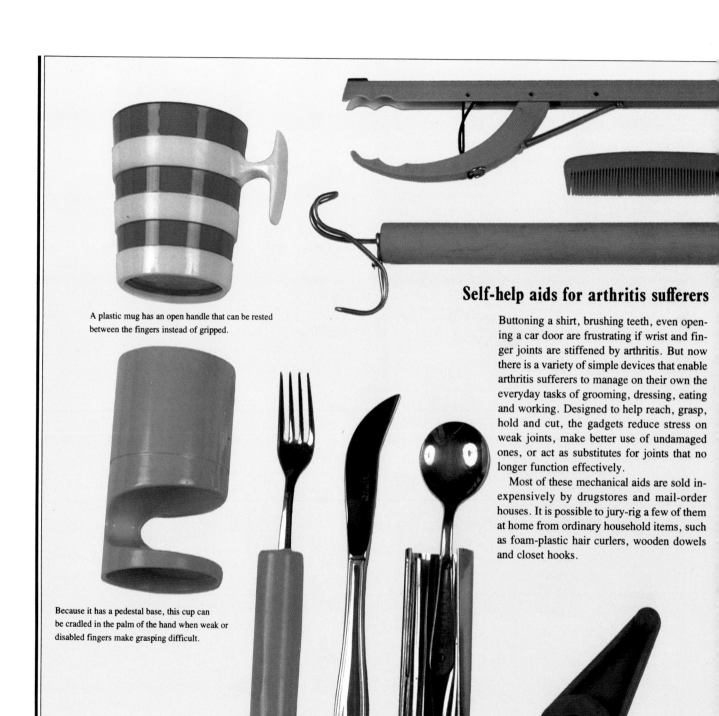

A plastic mug has an open handle that can be rested between the fingers instead of gripped.

Because it has a pedestal base, this cup can be cradled in the palm of the hand when weak or disabled fingers make grasping difficult.

Self-help aids for arthritis sufferers

Buttoning a shirt, brushing teeth, even opening a car door are frustrating if wrist and finger joints are stiffened by arthritis. But now there is a variety of simple devices that enable arthritis sufferers to manage on their own the everyday tasks of grooming, dressing, eating and working. Designed to help reach, grasp, hold and cut, the gadgets reduce stress on weak joints, make better use of undamaged ones, or act as substitutes for joints that no longer function effectively.

Most of these mechanical aids are sold inexpensively by drugstores and mail-order houses. It is possible to jury-rig a few of them at home from ordinary household items, such as foam-plastic hair curlers, wooden dowels and closet hooks.

Utensils for eating include a fork with built-up plastic handle for easy gripping, a knife that cuts by rocking instead of sawing and a spoon whose handle can be expanded so that it will fit the grasp.

A rubber tube fits over and extends door or faucet handles to give greater leverage.

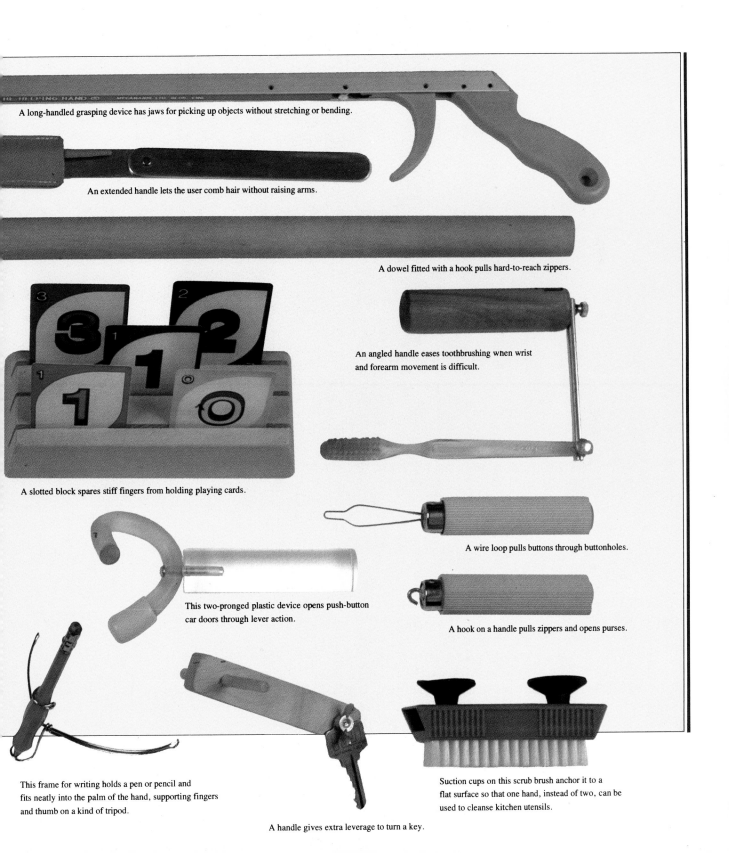

A long-handled grasping device has jaws for picking up objects without stretching or bending.

An extended handle lets the user comb hair without raising arms.

A dowel fitted with a hook pulls hard-to-reach zippers.

An angled handle eases toothbrushing when wrist and forearm movement is difficult.

A slotted block spares stiff fingers from holding playing cards.

A wire loop pulls buttons through buttonholes.

This two-pronged plastic device opens push-button car doors through lever action.

A hook on a handle pulls zippers and opens purses.

This frame for writing holds a pen or pencil and fits neatly into the palm of the hand, supporting fingers and thumb on a kind of tripod.

Suction cups on this scrub brush anchor it to a flat surface so that one hand, instead of two, can be used to cleanse kitchen utensils.

A handle gives extra leverage to turn a key.

A cauliflower-shaped white blood cell, part of the body's natural defense against disease, is pictured below, greatly magnified, as it attacks joint fibers. This process may cause arthritis: Joints swell with aroused white blood cells and delicate fibers are permanently damaged by chemicals the cells release.

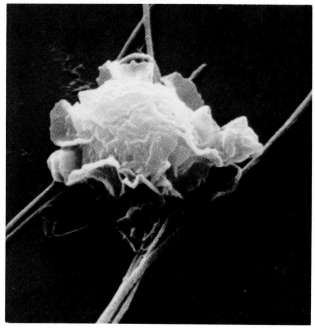

the arid desert of North Africa or Arizona. This is not necessarily true; generally as many residents of warm, sunny regions suffer as do those who live in the cold and damp.

Still, it is true that the aches and pains that accompany arthritis are less bothersome in warm, dry weather, as demonstrated in tests at the University of Pennsylvania. There Dr. Joseph L. Hollander asked a number of arthritis patients—two at a time—to spend two to four weeks living in a controlled-climate chamber. Without knowing what actually was being investigated, the patients kept detailed records of their fluid consumption, weight, temperature, joint stiffness, pain and the kind and amount of medicine they needed to curb the discomfort. What Dr. Hollander proved came as no surprise; the patients felt more pain and stiffness when the humidity rose and the barometric pressure dropped—just as many people do before it rains.

The reason for this adverse reaction to weather may be linked to shifting bodily fluids. To maintain equilibrium with the environment, the body's tissues respond to lowering atmospheric pressure by pushing out into the bloodstream either excess fluid or excess salts that hold fluid in the tissues. But joint tissues swollen or scarred by arthritis, theorized Dr. Hollander, cannot rid themselves of these excess fluids as promptly as normal tissues; liquid pressure in such tissue increases, relative to falling air pressure, and the result is a stiff, aching joint.

Another catalyst for rheumatoid arthritis is emotional stress. Although most specialists feel psychological strain is not the fundamental cause, they agree that it can worsen the symptoms, confirming the observation of the sufferer who reported, ''When I run up against a dead end I'm emotionally distraught, and my arthritis gets bad.''

Today, most experts believe the disease actually arises from infection, because the total pattern of rheumatoid arthritis symptoms has all the earmarks of an infectious illness, including fever, fatigue and aching muscles. Furthermore, an infection might also trigger a devastating malfunction of the immune system of the kind that is believed to cause arthritis. This system, the body's indispensable defense against invasion by enemies such as bacteria and viruses, marshals a powerful army of cells.

Composing one battalion of these cells are white blood cells of a type known as lymphocytes, which manufacture antibodies, the immune system's most sophisticated killers. The antibodies disarm an invader—or antigen, as invading substances are called when they set off antibodies—by latching onto its surface, blocking the attachment sites that enable an antigen to hook onto and infiltrate a healthy cell in the joint. The antigen is then no longer able to destroy the healthy cell. Instead the neutralized invader and the antibody now attached to it will combine with a blood substance called complement, forming a three-part complex that is a target for another battalion of white blood cells, scavengers called macrophages, literally ''big eaters.'' They swallow and digest the antigen-antibody-complement units; each big eater can devour as many as 100 invader particles.

But it appears that in rheumatoid arthritis and some other kinds of arthritis the defense system is sabotaged by a virus or some other infectious invader. Then the body's lymphocytes produce antibodies that, instead of attacking the invader, attack the cells of the joints' synovial membrane, provoking inflammation. The big eaters get their signals crossed, too, and, weakened somehow by the complexes they have eaten, they spill their digestive compounds into the joints' lubricating fluids. This poisoned fluid erodes the joint membrane, the spongy cartilage and, given enough time, the bone itself. As more misled lymphocytes and big eaters join the hostilities, what began as a campaign against a foreign invader turns into a crippling civil war.

The provocateur of this self-destruction is today thought to be some common virus that is carried by most people without harm, but that sometimes stirs itself into harmful action. One suspect is the Epstein-Barr virus, named after the British scientists who isolated it, which causes the ''kissing disease,'' infectious mononucleosis. Supporting evidence implicating Epstein-Barr virus has been uncovered by researchers at the University of California at San Diego, who discovered that rheumatoid arthritis sufferers have greater than normal amounts of this virus in their saliva.

Hereditary factors also may make some individuals more vulnerable to the kind of immune-system breakdown that seems involved in rheumatoid and other forms of arthritis. Studies of a group of 12 families by researchers from the University of Texas and the University of Alabama found, for example, that a genetic defect apparently permitted the parents to pass on to their children a susceptibility to rheumatoid arthritis. They discovered in some a ''genetic marker'' that identifies them as more likely than others to contract rheumatoid arthritis. The marker is an immune-system antigen known as DR4; it showed up in 65 per cent of all rheumatoid arthritis victims and in only 20 per cent of those people who do not suffer from the disease.

Whatever initially provokes rheumatoid arthritis, its vicious cycle of inflammation and stiffening—if allowed to continue unchecked—brings joint damage that eventually becomes irreversible. Under attack by the immune system, cells in the tissue of the joints explode and spill their chemical contents into the joint, where they cause more cell damage. As blood rushes in to repair the harm, blood vessels enlarge, producing swelling that squeezes and harms surrounding tis-

sues. Tiny blood clots may form within the vessels, blocking the healing blood supply without reducing pressures and swelling. If this inflammatory process is not interrupted, the damage spreads.

Inevitable trouble from wear and tear

This cycle of inflammation, pain and joint damage is the hallmark of rheumatoid arthritis, and the focus of its many-faceted treatment. But curiously, the most widespread form of arthritis—the word itself means inflammation of the joint—involves little or no inflammation. It is osteoarthritis, also called degenerative joint disease, in which the joints just stiffen up. The cartilage on the ends of the joint bones becomes pitted, frayed or worn away. As the cushioning cartilage disappears, the ends of the bones may grow lateral projections—spurs—perhaps to help spread the load on the joint and reduce the pressure of friction. But the spurs can themselves be a cause of danger and eventual harm. They may limit movement and stiffen the joint; they may also grate on one another and cause pain. In rare cases they may fuse the joint solid, particularly in the spine. The stiffening does not spread from joint to joint; its effect is limited to the few joints it may strike, and it is accompanied by no fever and no general feeling of misery.

Because osteoarthritis seems to be caused mainly by wear and tear—the repeated friction of the parts inside the joint—

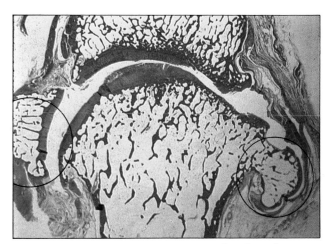

A stained cross section of a finger joint reveals arthritic bone spurs (circled). The spurs were the body's attempt to compensate for arthritis-damaged cartilage (blue tint) by broadening the area of contact between the two bone ends. Where the cartilage is actually missing, as at right, bone rubbed painfully against bone.

it can develop not only in older people but in anyone who subjects the joints to special stress: athletes, factory workers, carpenters or ballet dancers. Anyone over the age of 35, in fact, is likely to have at least a touch of osteoarthritis, although in most people the symptoms of the disease do not appear until the sixties and seventies. Perhaps in as much as a fourth of the total population it might be detected by X-rays of the joints, but many of these people do not even suspect that they have it.

Destruction of cartilage can occur in any joint that was defective at birth or subjected to later abuse. One manifestation of osteoarthritis is bony knobs on the end joints of the fingers, known as Heberden's nodes for the 18th Century British physician who first described them. These may develop in certain people, mainly women, who are predisposed by heredity to some sort of chemical change in their joint cartilage or synovial fluid.

But age and physical injury seem to be the principal causes of osteoarthritis. An accident that harms a joint might be to blame, or excess weight that overloads hips and knees, or repeated stresses from sports. Sometimes a series of injuries to the surrounding muscles or ligaments ends up injuring the joint itself. Once, a number of Canadian football players were examined and X-rayed by an arthritis study group and compared with a group of young men who were not professional athletes. Among the nonathletes, only 4 per cent showed some signs of osteoarthritis, while every one of the football players exhibited evidence of it. In addition to abuse from too-strenuous activities, such simple mechanical problems as poor posture or flat feet can damage the joints, because they throw the frame out of alignment and put harmful stresses on hips and knees.

Osteoarthritis may be crippling. The stereotypical victim is the old man with joints so stiffened he hobbles with a cane. But its signs are not always so obvious. Occasionally, nerves will be impaired if bone spurs press against them. One elderly woman suddenly found that her legs would collapse under her, causing her to sit down abruptly on the floor; doctors discovered that her spinal arthritis was momentarily numbing the nerves to and from her legs. A rheumatologist recalled

being consulted by two dentists who, by coincidence, were both suffering from an inability to hold and control a drill. Each thought he had arthritis in the hand. Instead both had osteoarthritis of the upper spine that temporarily deadened nerves from the neck. When they adopted a simple course of exercises for their necks, the pressure on the nerves was relieved and sensation returned.

The diet connection in gout

The characteristic cartilage breakdown and stiffness of osteoarthritis and other forms of arthritis are often laid to diet. Blamed are a lack of certain vitamins or of oil-rich foods that are believed to lubricate the joints, as if they were rusty hinges. One best-selling author claimed that arthritis sufferers benefit from an emulsion of cod liver oil and orange juice. Others have touted the preventive powers of such foods as alfalfa, blackstrap molasses, vinegar and honey. But scientists at both the Arthritis Foundation and the National Institute of Arthritis, Metabolism, and Digestive Diseases insist that diet has nothing to do with causing—or curing—any form of arthritis, the one exception being gout.

Long known as "the king of diseases and the disease of kings," gout was widely assumed to be just retribution for men who overindulged in wine, women and rich foods—diet was often seen as the sole cause. When the Maoris of New Zealand, who had subsisted on fish and vegetables, came under British influence and began eating beef, milk, bread and sugar, their incidence of both heart disease and gout increased rapidly.

Indeed, gout often stems from an inability—probably inherited—to process various foodstuffs adequately, leading to an excess of uric-acid wastes. Either overproduction or underexcretion of these wastes, or a combination of both, can lead to an attack of gout.

When susceptible individuals encourage overproduction of wastes by eating certain organ meats—kidneys, sweetbreads, liver—their bodies cannot handle the large amounts of uric acid that digestion of these foods produces. The excess uric acid that builds up in the body solidifies to form needle-like crystals in the joints. In other individuals, however, choice of food has little or nothing to do with gout; even when these people are put on a strict diet, their bodies produce too little or too much of certain enzymes that regulate the body's production of uric acid. Still others develop gout when their uric-acid levels are elevated by medical treatment—the "water pills" used for high blood pressure may so increase the loss of fluids that the body begins to reabsorb some wastes that would ordinarily be excreted, and in doing so holds onto uric acid.

The crystals from this acid engender inflammation that causes joints to become swollen, tender and incredibly painful—the big toe is hit first in three out of four victims. "If one of your friends," goes an old joke, "took a large pair of pliers and squeezed the big toe joint hard—that's arthritis. But if one of your enemies did it, then that's gout."

Today this type of arthritis is quickly and completely controllable—more so than any other chronic form. Usually a patient is first given colchicine, a powerful substance that comes from the autumn crocus, or colchicum plant. "I find the power of colchicum so great," the 19th Century English clergyman and wit Sydney Smith hyperbolized, "that if I feel a little gout coming on, I go into the garden, and hold out my toe to that plant, and it gets well directly." Colchicine is not quite as magical as the Reverend Smith claimed, but taken as a pill or injection, it relieves pain and swelling. It does not, however, lower the body's uric-acid levels and eliminate the cause of gout. So the victim may then be put on drugs such as probenecid or sulfinpyrazone, which help flush uric acid out through the kidneys, or on allopurinol, which inhibits uric-acid production.

When quick treatment counts

The sudden and unrelenting pain of gout will usually send its victim in search of a physician within days, if not hours. But the often episodic nature of rheumatoid arthritis or the gradual stiffening of osteoarthritis leads many sufferers to wait a while and see if the discomfort goes away. After all, commented one arthritis specialist, "not all joint aches point to arthritis. Most of us get minor aches and pains all the time, but they go away."

A medical mystery's artistic solution

Some forms of arthritis are indubitably ancient, recognizable in dinosaur bones and the mummies of Egyptian pharaohs. No such evidence of antiquity exists for the worst type of the disease, rheumatoid arthritis. First documented in Europe in 1800, it was considered a new ailment, resulting from the change to an industrialized society.

But after examining paintings of the 17th Century Flemish master Peter Paul Rubens, Belgian and American experts concluded in 1977 that the artist—and some of his subjects—probably had rheumatoid arthritis. In his late works, such as the self-portrait below, many subjects display the enlarged wrists and fingers of the disease, suggesting that it is at least 160 years older than previously thought.

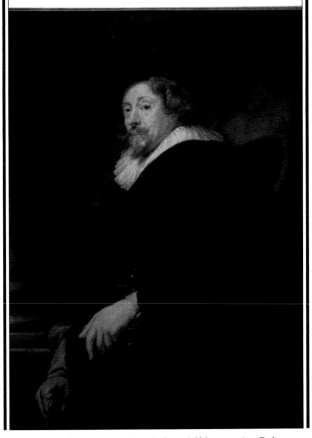

In his last self-portrait, painted about 1639, an aging Rubens painstakingly detailed the rheumatoid deformities and swelling of his left hand. The ailing artist relied on a sword, barely visible under his crippled hand, as a walking stick.

Pain in or near the joints could be due to simple muscle strain *(Chapter 4)* or to bursitis *(page 91),* the inflammation of the protective sacs around the joint; both conditions respond to such simple treatment as aspirin, rest and cold packs. Within six weeks the natural healing process usually has taken care of most nonarthritic aches. "Treat yourself the way you would instruct a child who doesn't feel well," advised Dr. Harry Spiera. "Get plenty of sleep, keep warm, avoid strenuous activity."

However, these measures of home treatment may not suffice. If pain persists daily, if stiffness and swelling continue, or if there is any tingling sensation at the end of a limb, it is important to see a doctor and have the condition diagnosed: Long delay compounds the damage, and the varied types of arthritis may call for differing treatments.

Diagnosis is a process of elimination. Excluding, one by one, the ailments that might have produced the patient's symptoms, the doctor narrows down the possibilities. For example, a patient might report the following symptoms: pain without inflammation, stiffness increasing throughout the day in only certain afflicted joints, and perhaps some disability but no fever or fatigue. This pattern of symptoms would not necessarily confirm osteoarthritis, but it would point a doctor away from a diagnosis of rheumatoid arthritis, which is usually characterized by more severe, overall symptoms and often symmetry of afflicted joints. Pain in a toe joint may suggest gout.

After the initial physical examination and interview, the doctor may order X-rays and also various laboratory tests. The lab tests are usually more helpful in making the original diagnosis; X-rays can help confirm a diagnosis, but because changes in cartilage or bones may not be visible in the early months of the disease, the X-ray photographs tend to be more useful as a kind of baseline for measuring later damage, should it occur. To survey the inside of a joint at an earlier stage, the doctor might scrutinize it with an arthroscope, the device that is most frequently used to examine sprained knees *(pages 96-107).*

Analysis of the fluid in a joint may also help determine the kind of arthritis a patient has. The fluid can be removed quite simply and relatively painlessly by tapping a joint with a hypodermic syringe. In rare instances where bacteria such as gonococcus or staphylococcus could be the direct cause of infectious arthritis, small pieces of inflamed joint tissue may be removed for examination under a microscope to search for an organism.

A doctor also does routine blood tests to check for elevated uric-acid levels, a sign of gout, and to see if there are more than the normal number of white blood cells in circulation. When rheumatoid arthritis is in an acute stage, the white-cell count may be up. But a more revealing blood test is the test done to look for the "rheumatoid factor," an antibody that turns up in the blood of 80 per cent of rheumatoid-arthritis victims. Some experts think this antibody may help fight disease and others think it may be a reaction to sickness. Whichever is the case, the doctor can use it as a clue—but only as a single clue in a pattern of evidence. He cannot diagnose rheumatoid arthritis because the rheumatoid factor is present or exclude the disease because it is absent.

A further clue may come from measuring the blood's sedimentation rate—the speed with which red blood cells settle to the bottom of a test tube. The more inflamed the joint affected by rheumatoid arthritis, the faster the red cells drop. In any inflammatory condition such as rheumatoid arthritis, there is an increase in blood protein that causes the red blood cells to stick together; their combined weight then makes them sink more quickly.

Aided by such tests, the doctor can usually pinpoint the problem. If the diagnosis is gout, the treatment is simple and direct. If the illness is either of the other most common types, osteoarthritis or rheumatoid arthritis, the physician and the patient will have reached a kind of fork in the road where two different paths of treatment branch off. The treatments are similar, but because rheumatoid arthritis is so complex its management is decidedly more complicated.

For both osteoarthritis and rheumatoid arthritis, most doctors today prescribe not one remedy but several. Medication to reduce swelling, pain and any inflammation will be at the core of the program, and the drugs prescribed may range from relatively innocuous substances such as aspirin to steroids that powerfully affect bodily processes. In addition, rest and exercise are standard recommendations. Most doctors will prescribe more rest and less exercise early in treatment—to allow swelling and inflammation to decrease. Later the patient is encouraged to perform gentle exercises that put joints through their full range of motion, not ones that pound on joints and provoke inflammation. Many activities suggested for healthy people, such as taking the stairs instead of the elevator, can actually increase arthritic inflammation and tissue damage.

The kinds of exercise doctors prescribe for those with arthritis involve smooth motions like those of swimming. The buoyancy of water confers a great benefit by helping to support the body and allowing movement at any pace that is comfortable. Some arthritis sufferers believe that swimming alone has enabled them to master the disease. One severely crippled woman recovered sufficiently to drive her car and even go on hikes: "My muscles used to get so tense and aching when I got cold," she said. "Then to ease into this water—from the first time I just knew it was the right thing for me." Another swimmer emphasized that her water exercises were effective only if she did them unstintingly. Once she took a leisurely vacation in California, visiting relatives and relaxing, but omitting her daily swim. As the weeks passed, she said, "I felt stiffer and tighter throughout my body. I also had slight pains in my neck and hands." She returned to New York and after a week of exercising in water, she was "back to normal."

Lightweight splints or braces, usually worn just while sleeping, may also be prescribed for resting and protecting damaged joints. Cold packs to reduce swelling may be part of the early treatment; in later stages of therapy, hot packs, hot baths and sometimes paraffin wax treatments *(page 149)* are used to increase circulation and restore ease of movement in stiffened joints.

Making sound choices from an arsenal of drugs

Most of these treatments are recommended for all arthritis victims. The medication prescribed is not so standardized, however, because every person's system handles drugs in a different manner. Countless arthritis sufferers never require any other kind of medicine than aspirin, which works amazingly well in reducing inflammation and curbing pain. But to be effective against arthritis, aspirin must be taken in great quantity, and in such large amounts it can produce harmful side effects.

Should aspirin fail, the physician usually tries one of the several relatively new anti-inflammation drugs, such as fenoprofen, ibuprofen, indomethacin or sulindac. Like aspirin, these drugs apparently work by preventing the release of inflammation-producing substances called prostaglandins. A more dangerous drug of the same class, phenylbutazone, or bute, is used occasionally for relieving symptoms of rheumatoid arthritis but is primarily used for short-term treatments of ankylosing spondylitis or gout. It can produce such severe side effects as high fever and the slowing down of blood formation in the bone marrow.

Another family of drugs, based on the malaria medicine quinine, brings relief to some rheumatoid-arthritis patients who are not helped by the anti-inflammation drugs. This group of drugs is believed to work by stabilizing the enzyme-containing sacs in the scavenger cells of the body's immune system. Once medication is initiated, signs of improvement may take only a month to appear, but the patient must be checked regularly for any eye problems that might develop—in rare instances the drug can accumulate in the retina and cause blindness.

Two other major arthritis drugs—different in name and nature but strikingly similar in their results—are gold and penicillamine, a nonantibiotic cousin of penicillin. In England penicillamine pills are often tried first, in the United States gold injections. The nature of penicillamine's action has not been established. It may not reduce inflammation, kill cells or suppress the immune system. Instead, it is theorized that the drug reduces the number of immune complexes—those antibody-antigen-blood complement bundles that in a normal person would be digested by the scavenging big eaters of the immune system, but in a person with arthritis might get into the joint fluid and begin destroying tissue. Penicillamine also may stabilize joint membranes so as to

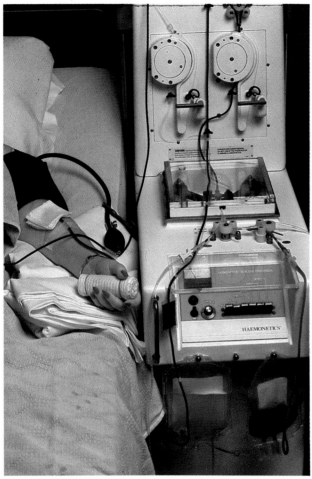

Blood from a vein in the arm of an arthritis patient is processed in this machine, which removes presumably harmful components, then returns what is left through a tube in the other arm.
Working like a cream separator, the device spins blood to separate its parts by weight, discarding into one plastic bag straw-colored plasma, the lightest ingredient, and into the other, heavier white blood cells (the white-cell bag is colored red by the presence of a few red cells). In trials at Los Angeles' Cedars-Sinai Medical Center, eliminating these two components helped some rheumatoid-arthritis victims—but researchers are not sure why.

prevent these immune complexes from setting off a cycle of destruction.

Unlike penicillamine, the gold salts appear to directly suppress an immune system gone awry. The gold may prevent sacs inside the big eaters from dumping out the destructive chemicals that harm joint tissue and signal the big eaters to attack normal cells. The gold also may inhibit the growth and proliferation of defending white blood cells—lymphocytes —that have turned against body tissues.

The effectiveness of gold compounds was discovered in the 1920s by a French physician, Dr. Jacques Forestier, who thought rheumatoid arthritis resembled tuberculosis, for which gold was then prescribed. To his amazement and that of doctors ever since, the substance not only reduced the inflammation of rheumatoid arthritis but in some cases promoted remission of the disease.

Gold salts are reduced to powder form, then combined with other chemicals and either water or oil in 1 to 10 per cent solutions; given by weekly injection, they are a mainstay of long-term therapy for many people: 70 per cent of those who receive them exhibit measurable improvement. But others cannot tolerate the side effects the gold solution shares with penicillamine: skin rash, ulcers in the mouth, diarrhea and, more worrisome, damage to the kidneys and to the blood-manufacturing bone marrow.

Despite such complications, these medicines are widely accepted; there are others, however, whose potency and dangerous side effects raise controversy. One is the industrial solvent dimethyl sulfoxide, or DMSO, which is sometimes applied to the skin to reduce the inflammation of strains and sprains *(Chapter 4)*, and is being tested on arthritis. Similarly controversial medicines are the immunosuppressives first used in cancer chemotherapy. Such powerful compounds as azathioprine and cyclophosphamide restrain the immune system from warring against body tissues, as it may do in rheumatoid arthritis. But in the process, they might render the suppressed immune system incapable of defending the body, so doctors are reluctant to prescribe them except in advanced cases.

Like the immunosuppressives, the powerful corticosteroids—synthetic versions of the inflammation-suppressing hormones manufactured by the body's adrenal glands—have been surrounded by controversy almost since the day of their introduction. In 1949 the news of the first of them, cortisone, seemed too good to be true: An arthritic patient hospitalized with stiff swollen joints and virtually unable to get out of bed was given an injection of the new drug; three days later she arose and walked with barely a limp. A few days after that she was out of the hospital, happily shopping. When one of the drug's creators, Dr. Philip Hench of the Mayo Clinic, reported his findings to a medical convention, the normally staid audience stood up and cheered.

Then came the bad news. Heavy, protracted use could lead to ulcers, bacterial infections, cataracts, fragile bones, excessive facial hair and a peculiar redistribution of body fat: Fat is eliminated from the body's extremities, only to collect at the back of the neck, forming "buffalo humps," and in the face, giving a moon-faced look.

Corticosteroids may also cause the hormone-producing adrenal glands to malfunction. When a person takes the synthetic, the body reacts just as if it had revved up its own production of hormones. The medicine will improve metabolism, reduce inflammation, restrain the destructive activity of lymphocytes, and even help release the brain's natural painkillers, known as endorphins. However, if these drugs are supplied in large doses over a long period of time, the adrenal glands may cut down production of natural cortisone and, should the dosage then be cut back or stopped, the body is left unprotected. The result may be fever, low blood pressure and, in some cases, even death. "Cortisone," recalled one authority, "became the model of a drug that provides early benefits but late penalties."

Today many physicians feel that cortisone and its equivalents, taken orally, are still worth prescribing—if only in small doses—because their sensational short-term effects may do much good before the long-term side effects develop. The steroids appear particularly helpful to lupus victims, for whom treatment of a severe flare-up may be lifesaving. Other physicians are loath to use steroids for any ailment besides lupus, except as a last resort.

The injection of cortisone directly into a joint is common but also somewhat controversial. Because the effect is localized, the injections appear to be less dangerous. What is more, the results can be wonderfully swift. One woman who had been unable to push the button that opened her car door was given an injection in her hand and the following day could open the door easily.

One or another of these medicines—from aspirin to cortisone—helps a great many people, but according to one leading rheumatologist, at least 20 per cent of arthritis sufferers are not relieved by any of them. So the disappointed continue to search for a cure, often turning to untested remedies. Said one patient, "When you have had that much pain you get so you'll try anything."

From mystical medicines to copper bracelets

Many victims do try anything—and become the willing targets of quacks and frauds. For every dollar spent on arthritis research, reported one survey, 25 are spent on unproven nostrums, worthless food supplements and "miracle cures." But none of the secret Indian medicines, magic horse collars or sure-cure diet books is worth anything, in the opinion of arthritis experts. Noted an official publication of the U.S. Food and Drug Administration, "You can hang a Vryllium tube on your lapel, bury yourself up to the neck in horse manure, swill Dr. Fenby's Formula X, or take a dose of 'Chuei-Fong-Tou-Geu-Wan,' but you will not be able to cure your arthritis."

Although responsible physicians condemn such treatments as wasteful and potentially harmful, business continues to be brisk. Former professional athlete Jerry Walsh, who suffered from rheumatoid arthritis, once made a television appearance on behalf of the Arthritis Foundation to display and denounce a number of sure-cure hoaxes. The station was deluged with calls—from viewers wanting to know where they could buy the objects.

Purveyors of such items cite names of persons who have been cured. That they can do so with veracity is due to the same quirk that makes arthritis so elusive: its capacity for suddenly vanishing, for going into spontaneous remission.

Patients experiencing such blessed relief are easily persuaded they owe it all to the most recent nostrum they tried. Somehow the public never hears about the legions of sufferers whom the device did not benefit—or those whom it may actually have harmed.

The injury that arthritis quacks can inflict is serious. One "secret medicine" sold by a Canadian practitioner turned out to be a hazardous blend of sex hormones and other endocrine drugs. Other "miracle" pills, passed off as perfectly safe, have turned out to contain indiscriminate amounts of powerful corticosteroids among their dangerous ingredients. Such pills, said one rheumatologist, give "days of relief and years of consequences"; many users in fact have died. One 61-year-old Illinois farmer, given pills a practitioner claimed were "only herbs . . . they will take your pain away," collapsed four hours later in his motel room. Rushed to a nearby hospital, he bled to death. The examining physician unequivocally blamed the pills, noting on the death certificate that the bleeding had been swiftly brought about by "ulcer due to cortisone."

Mercifully, no harm is inflicted by one of the most popular of the magical treatments for arthritis, the copper bracelet. There is no evidence that this amulet confers any physical benefit; for one thing, metallic copper cannot be absorbed through the skin. But many arthritis sufferers claim to have been helped by it.

The copper bracelet's alleged powers seem to be derived from the practice of Romans who, 2,000 years ago, visited

An Old-World remedy: mud baths

Every year, in a ritual dating back to the Fifth Century B.C., thousands of people suffering from arthritis and rheumatism descend on commercial spas in the little Italian town of Abano Terme, near Venice, to have their aching joints and muscles packed and soothed in volcanic mud brought from nearby hot springs. Exactly how the mud works its supposedly therapeutic magic is the subject of debate. Its penetrating heat, exceeding 100°, undoubtedly has sedative effects, similar to those of the hot waxes employed in some American clinics *(page 149)*. Less perfectly understood are the purported contributions of the mud's mineral salts, natural radioactivity and algae, which flourish in the slimy broth.

Because of these uncertainties and the absence of objective proof of effectiveness, many physicians look askance at such mud therapy. But it is considered a safe and sometimes useful regimen by numbers of European and Middle Eastern rheumatologists, and mud therapy is under extensive study in the Soviet Union and Eastern Europe.

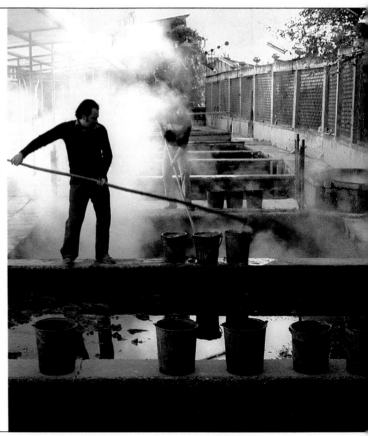

Buckets of steaming mud, ready for the treatment rooms, are filled from Abano Terme's concrete holding ponds, where the grayish-green mud matures for six months after it is dredged from nearby thermal pools. During that time, the rich mineral mix and heat foster the growth of tiny algae, which give the matured mud a uniquely soft and oily consistency.

the spa in Bath, England. After immersing themselves in the reputedly curative waters, sufferers—now feeling much better—indicated their gratitude by affixing to the wall by the waters of the public bath copper bracelets bearing their names, much as supplicants in more recent times have hung crutches at a shrine. Over the centuries the legend grew that Bath's waters, lapping at the bracelets, thereby gained extra potency. In more recent times, when electricity and copper wires came into use, the legend took on another facet: The bracelet, it was said, somehow conveyed harmful electricity away from the body.

The likeliest explanation for the bracelet's supposed efficacy is the placebo effect—the curative power of an inactive medicine given merely to satisfy a patient. If a patient thinks a placebo will work, it often does. Thus the copper bracelet may help precisely because the arthritis victim is convinced that it will.

How joints are repaired—or replaced

The psychological impact of a copper bracelet may lessen pain and stiffness, but it cannot make a joint destroyed by arthritis function again. Modern surgical techniques can. A pioneer in surgery to resurface arthritis-ravaged joints with healthy cartilage, Dr. Marvin Meyers of the University of Texas Southwestern Medical School, reported a success rate of 85 per cent in 50 operations; most patients were able to put their full weight on the repaired joints within six months.

Some less extensive operations, such as the removal of

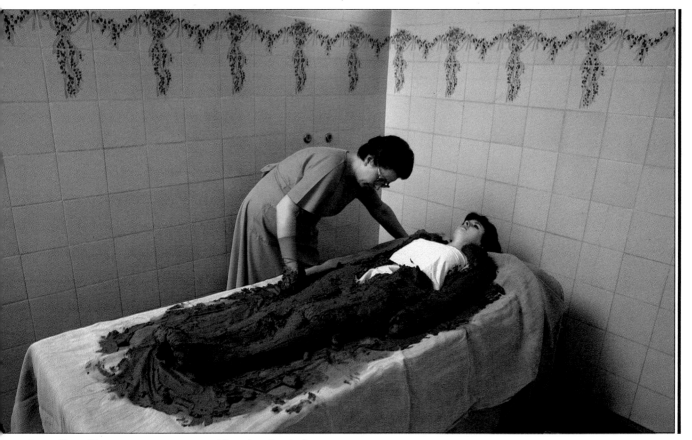

In an Abano Terme treatment room, a rubber-gloved attendant slathers 109° mud onto a patient in thick layers, leaving only her chest and head uncovered. Patients report that the treatment, which usually lasts 20 minutes, induces a drowsy euphoria as heat radiates throughout the body, followed by an hour or so of profuse perspiration once the mud is removed.

Steel and plastic replacements for frozen joints

Even if arthritis freezes a joint, making it almost immovable, a remedy is now at hand. The natural joint can be replaced with a synthetic one, made of stainless steel and plastic.

The first successful replacement, performed in the early 1960s by British surgeon John Charnley after two decades of experimentation, was a hip joint. Since then, replacement of joints with synthetic substitutes like those at right—not only hips but also knees, elbows, shoulders, wrists and fingers—has become a practical option for the millions who suffer the pain of disabling arthritis.

The most successful implants, however, have been those of the hip and knee. Large, weight-bearing joints, their movements are less complex, their structures less delicate than those of most other skeletal connections. In an average year, for example, 160,000 Americans are outfitted with artificial hips or knees; by contrast, a bare 20,000 people worldwide receive man-made shoulders. Yet lightweight, high-performance steel alloys of cobalt-chromium and the titanium used in spacecraft promise to make replacements for the most delicate joints—even the ankle, one of the body's most complex and highly stressed joints—increasingly feasible in the years ahead.

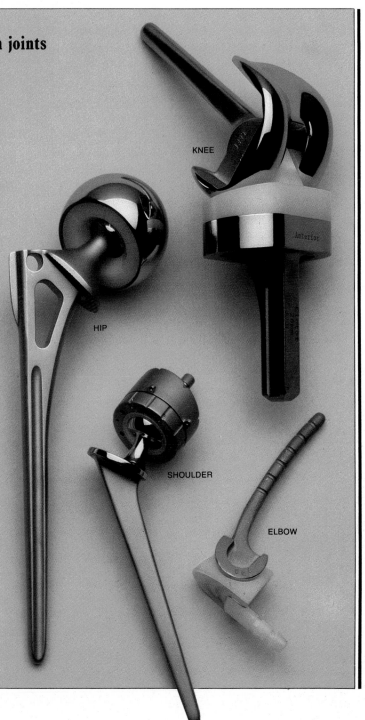

KNEE

HIP

SHOULDER

ELBOW

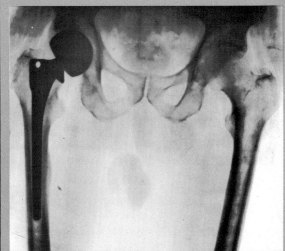

How closely man-made joints mimic nature's own is shown in this X-ray of the pelvis of an arthritis victim fitted with a hip joint (left) of metal and plastic. It is the type shown at right above, with three other common replacements.

inflamed synovial membrane, are now being done in certain hospitals with the help of a device called the arthroscope, which eliminates the need to cut open the entire joint. This instrument is the length of a drinking straw with an eyepiece (or television camera) at one end and at the other a light and a lens. Cutting instruments—all very tiny—can be threaded through the tube and controlled from the eyepiece end. The entire device is slender enough to be inserted into the joint, like a needle. Glass fibers inside the tube carry the lens's view of the joint's interior to the eye of the surgeon, who then manipulates the controls to cut away diseased membrane. In many cases the patient, with an incision only an inch long, can get out of bed and walk on his repaired joint the next day.

If a joint has been so badly damaged that it is useless, it now can be replaced with a man-made substitute, meticulously fashioned of metal and plastic to perform most of the same complex motions as the original. Twenty years after such an operation was first performed in the United States, 160,000 people a year were fitted there with artificial joints.

Of course, substitutes for human body parts—prostheses—are as old as the wooden leg, and even more complex types have been made for centuries. The 16th Century French surgeon, Ambroise Paré, devised numerous artificial hands, arms and legs of steel, some with moving parts. But such devices were additions to the body, strapped onto the outside—little help for an arthritic joint. Only in recent decades—as surgeons and scientists came up with a metal cup to fit into the pelvis and receive the head of the thighbone, and then a plastic replacement for the thighbone head—did a total joint replacement for inside the body become possible.

The artificial joints that now enable those crippled with arthritis to walk are largely the result of a quarter century of work by the British orthopedic specialist, Sir John Charnley. A major difficulty he encountered—and eventually overcame—was finding materials strong enough to withstand immense loads and absorb stress, and yet remain compatible with and uncorroded by the body's tissues and fluids. Finally, following World War II, two such materials became available: the plastic polyethylene, used for toys and food bags, and stainless steel. Sir John combined these to create a low-friction ball-and-socket joint for the hip. But how to hold it in place? He got his answer from a professor of dentistry who recommended the cement called methyl methacrylate, used to hold in fillings and fix dentures. Unfortunately, while the cement can last up to 25 years with normal use, it is not permanent. So work continues to find a better glue.

Today replacements are available for several joints. They mean a second chance at an active, normal life for many arthritis victims. A San Francisco woman in her late fifties had been bedridden with rheumatoid arthritis until operations replaced both her hips with artificial joints. Soon she was able to walk again; she returned to work and a busy social life. "I go up and down stairs," she said, "on and off street cars, everything." A New York lawyer, reduced to walking with two canes by osteoarthritis of his hip, finally decided to have the hip replaced. After surgery and six months of therapy, he was playing tennis—without even a limp. Even more dramatic was the joint-replacement surgery for a doctor who had long suffered from rheumatoid arthritis: Today he is busily engaged in his practice equipped with two new hips, two new knees, two new wrists and one new ankle.

Only a few of the many millions of arthritis sufferers require such drastic treatment as joint replacement. All require one essential kind of treatment that only they can provide: resolve. Said one former sufferer, "The most important thing is, don't despair. You must fight it. Don't give up."

A woman in her fifties, who had fought arthritis for some 30 years and had overcome it, put it another way. She and a friend had come down with the disease at the same time but, she recalled, "there was just one difference. She had lots of money and I didn't. As soon as she developed arthritis she began to feel sorry for herself. She spent the next ten years of her life, and much of her husband's money, going from doctor to doctor trying to find a sure cure. In addition, she had nurses to wait on her. It wasn't possible for me to do that, for I had to be out working every day, so I went to the doctor and told him, 'With your help and God's we're going to beat this.' I can't say we've beaten it entirely, but I've lost very few days from work, because I've kept after it and kept on my feet. I had to; she didn't." ✻

Taming the great crippler

Only a few of the many diseases called arthritis can be cured. But the crippling that once seemed an almost inevitable consequence of arthritis can often be treated by modern rehabilitation techniques that enable stiffened joints to function almost like new.

At hospitals specializing in arthritis, such as the Spain Rehabilitation Center at the University of Alabama, where the pictures on these and the following pages were taken, the restoration of arthritic joints usually involves not only drugs and surgery but also physical therapy and so-called occupational therapy.

Physical therapy seeks to restore motion and strength to large joints, principally in the hips and legs, so that a patient can walk in reasonable comfort. Heat treatments—many relying on water *(right)*—are used to relieve pain and stiffness. Gentle exercises put joints through their full range of motion, extending the range gradually. Therapists teach patients who cannot move on their own how to use canes and crutches to best effect.

Occupational therapy, despite its name, has less to do with a job than with everyday living—it prepares the joints of the arms and hands to manage buttons and keys. Therapists teach patients exercises to increase the strength and flexibility of arms, wrists, hands and fingers. In special workshops, patients learn how to perform everyday tasks without pain.

"Although all chronic arthritics have to accept some degree of discomfort and disability," said Dr. Bevra Hahn, Director of the Washington University National Institutes of Health Arthritis Center in St. Louis, "in all but the most severe cases, we can rehabilitate a patient."

Elizabeth Stubbs lies partially submerged in swirling warm water while a therapist gently bends her arm at the elbow. Relaxed and soothed by the water's heat, all of her arthritic joints will be exercised by the therapist to begin the process of restoring their ability to move.

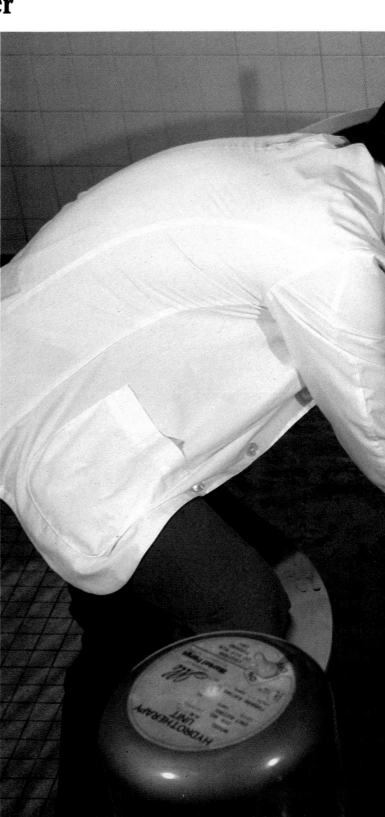

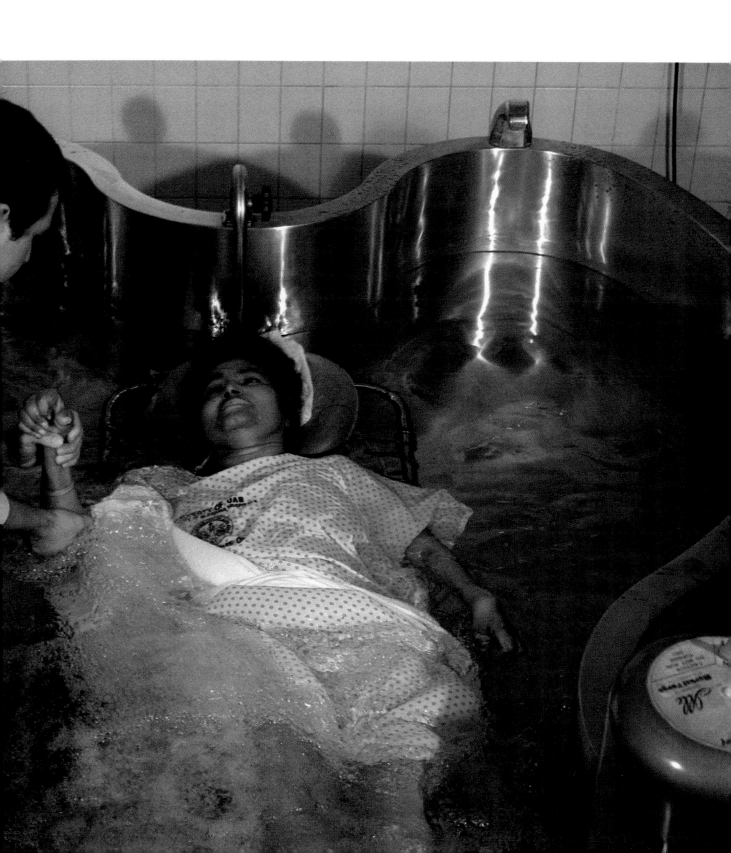

Physical therapy: regaining independence

Some arthritis patients arrive at a rehabilitation center in wheel-chairs or with joints virtually locked. After a week or more, many are able to leave on their feet, with motion in large joints restored.

The secret of such recovery is simple: about two hours a day of exercise, generally performed with a therapist's help in large, heated pools. The warmth speeds the healing of the inflamed tissues and soothes muscles and joints so that they can be moved easily, while the water's buoyancy supports the body and helps take weight off painful joints.

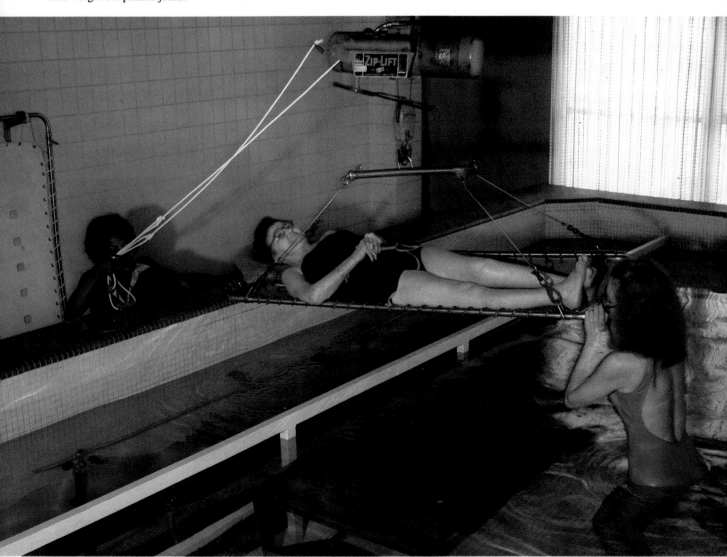

Resting on a stretcher attached to a motorized crane, Vera Drain is lowered onto a submerged table in a heated exercise pool by physical therapist Judi Parker (right) and an attendant. The patient, whose rheumatoid arthritis makes walking difficult, will lie motionless for a time, partly covered by the warm water, so that her joints and muscles loosen.

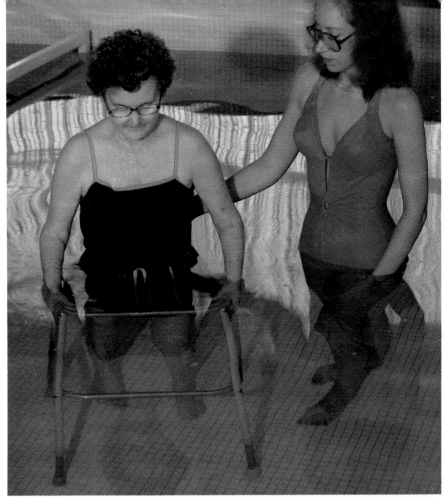

Judi Parker lends a helping hand as Vera Drain, now acclimated to the shallow, warm water, takes a few tentative steps aided by a four-legged walker that gives balance and support. Once she gains confidence walking in the pool, she will try it on land— first with the walker, then without.

The hands of an arthritis patient glisten with melted paraffin and mineral oil. The hands are dipped in the brew until eight to 12 layers are accumulated; then, glazed with hardened wax, they are wrapped in towels for 20 minutes to retain heat. The soothing effect of the warmth lasts for hours, allowing the patient to work without pain.

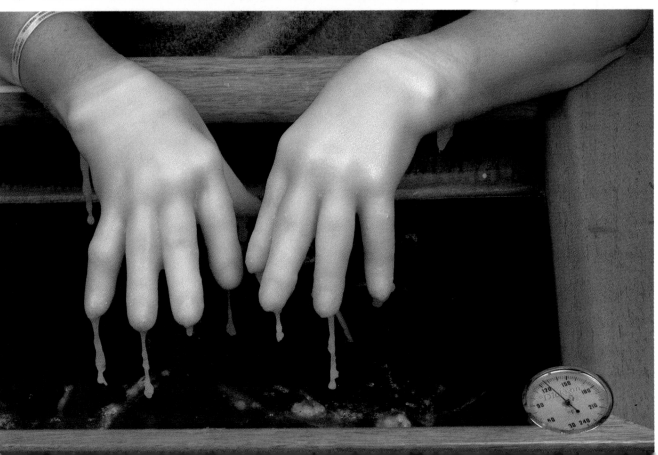

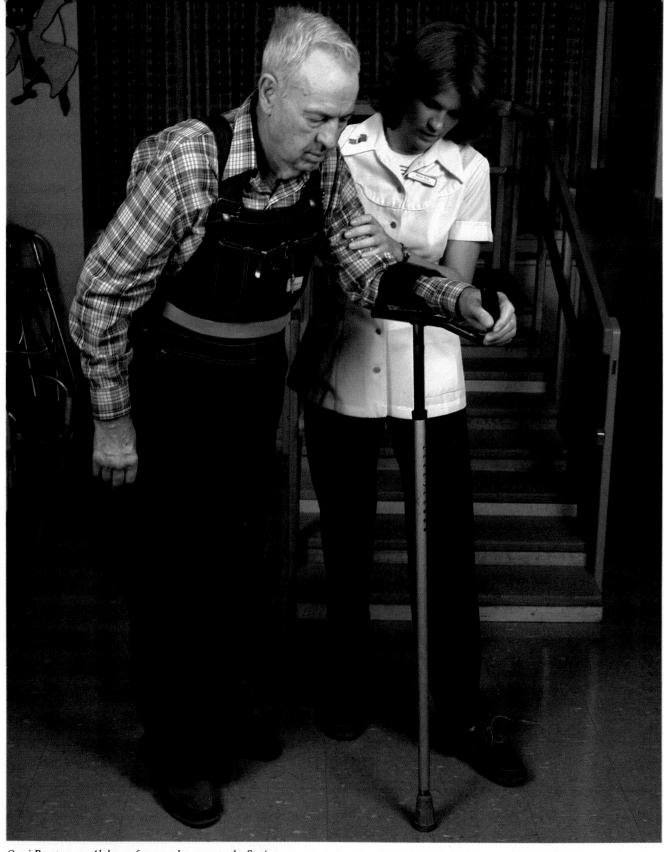

Omri Preston, an Alabama farmer who came to the Spain Center in a wheelchair, learns to walk again with a T-shaped crutch; it supports his weight on his forearm bones rather than on the more fragile bones of his hand and wrist, as a cane would. A therapist guides him and supports him by holding his belt.

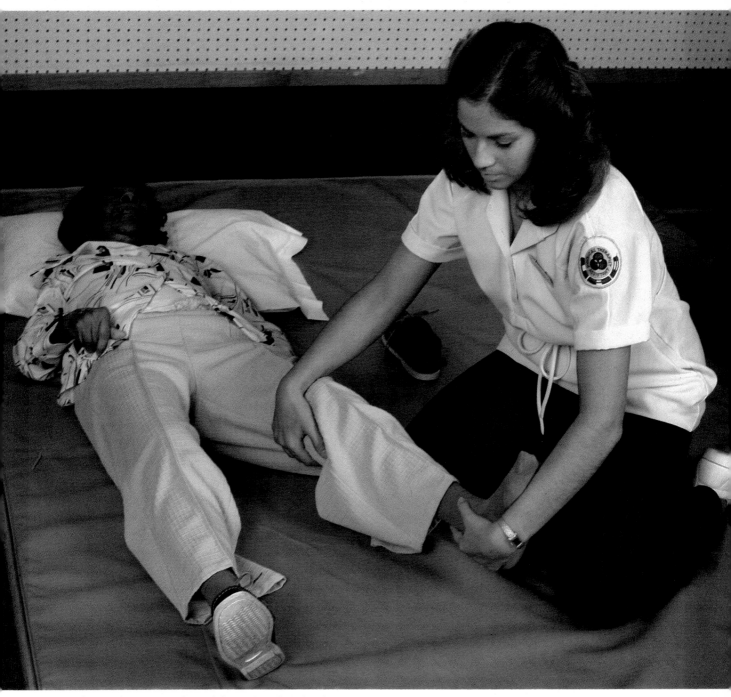

Marsha Roberson, a student in physical therapy, works to bend and extend the knee of Eva Moss, an arthritis patient. In this so-called passive exercise, joints and muscles are moved by the therapist without the patient's help; such movement prevents the crippling stiffness that can result from lack of use.

How much progress? How soon?

To see how arthritic joints respond to treatment, therapists check progress periodically with instruments that measure a patient's strength and range of motion. An arthritic's posture—checked simply by photographing the patient through a grid *(opposite)*—often discloses tight muscles or weak joints. If a patient seems to lean to one side, for example, it may indicate that a joint on that side has not strengthened as expected. "Almost everyone gains some improvement," said physical therapist Judi Parker.

If no progress is evident after two to six weeks—and if the therapists are sure a patient is working as hard as possible—the therapy itself may be changed. The frequency of heat treatments may be increased or decreased; exercise time in the pool may be augmented by exercises out of it; stretching exercises may be added to a regimen of bending and flexing the joints. Doctors may alter drug prescriptions. If surgery is required, it is followed by another course of physical therapy, often using modified exercises to restore movement and prevent weakness.

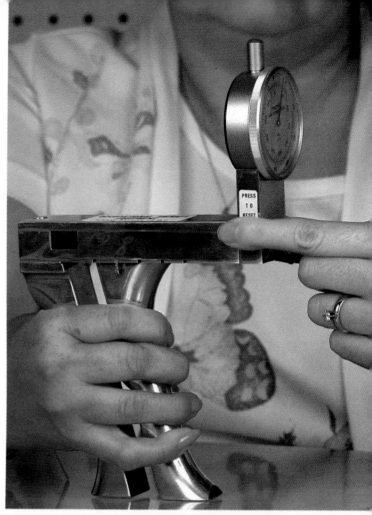

The stiffened fingers of a patient's right hand squeeze a gunlike dynamometer to test hand strength; a therapist's hand (right) steadies the device. This patient could exert a force of only 20 pounds (40 to 50 pounds would be normal for a woman of her age).

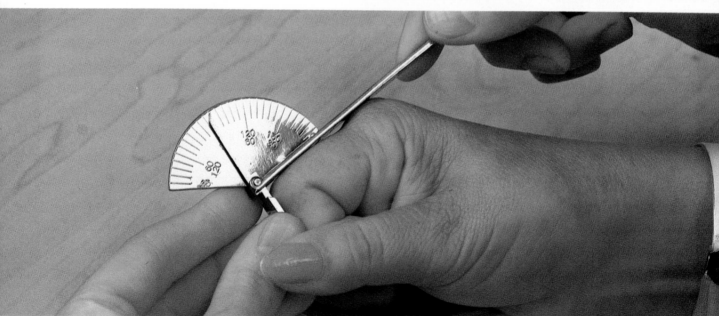

A device called a goniometer measures the angle formed by the index finger of a rheumatoid-arthritis patient who has made a fist. The angle—about 90°—is almost normal and shows a significant improvement since the start of the patient's therapy.

Maurice Halsey stands behind a clear plastic grid, its horizontal and vertical lines revealing how straight she can stand. A photograph like this was compared with one of the patient taken earlier. It proved what therapists had suspected—three weeks of intensive therapy allowed her to stand straighter.

Therapist Pam Porter uses a larger version of the angle-measuring goniometer in order to determine how far Maurice Halsey can extend her elbow joint. Because the patient is still unable to straighten her arm, she needs more therapy.

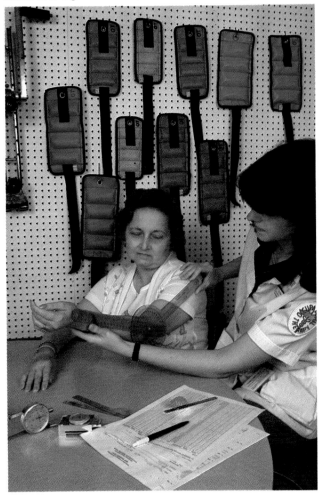

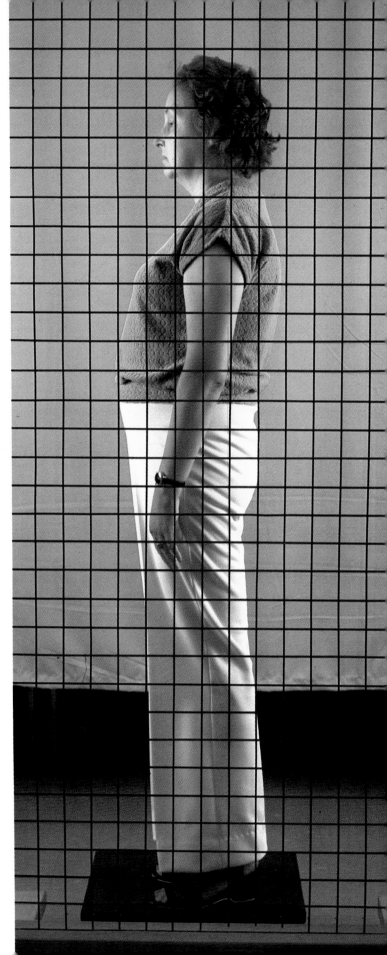

Therapy for the little things in life

It is life's little tasks—brushing teeth, fastening buttons, turning doorknobs—that often frustrate arthritis victims most. To do what stiffened fingers and partially immobilized shoulders or legs cannot, a number of specialized but simple gadgets are available—the most common are pictured on pages 132-133. At the Spain Center patients practice cooking, washing and dressing with mechaical aids adapted to their disabilities. But the major improvement in manipulative abilities must come from specific exercises in fine work *(following pages)*.

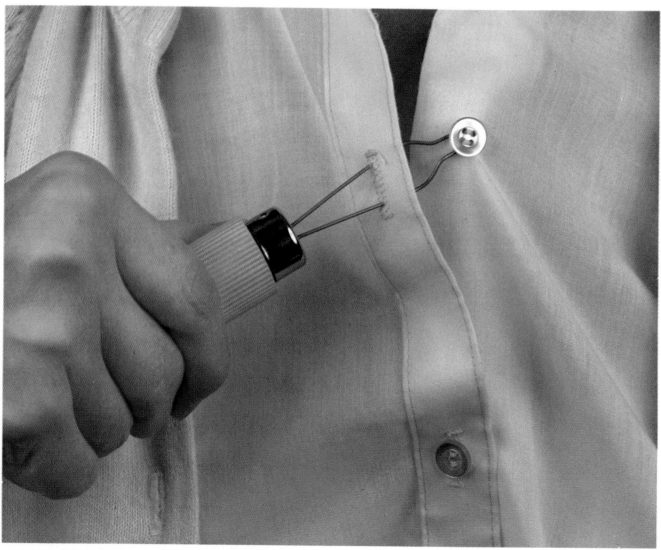

A woman with arthritic fingers uses a buttonhook to fasten her blouse: She first passes the wire loop through the buttonhole and over the button, then pulls back, drawing the button through the hole. The thick handle makes the tool easy to maneuver.

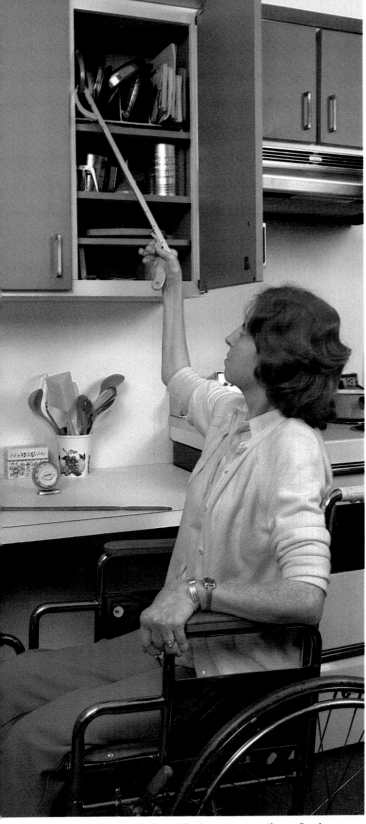

In a practice kitchen, Barbara Rhodes—temporarily confined to a wheelchair because of recent surgery to replace an arthritic knee—picks a potlid off a high shelf with a long-handled reacher. A trigger on the handle activates its grasping tongs.

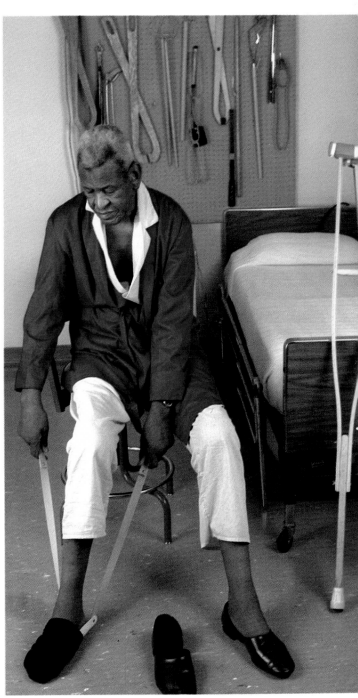

Recuperating from surgery that replaced his arthritic hip, James Thomas uses a stocking aid. He gathers the sock over a U-shaped frame. Then he slips his foot into the sock and pulls it up by the device's straps; the frame slips off over the heel.

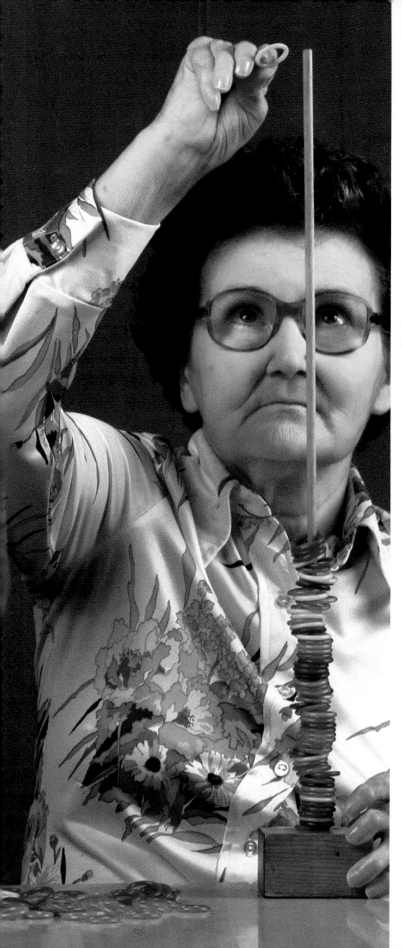

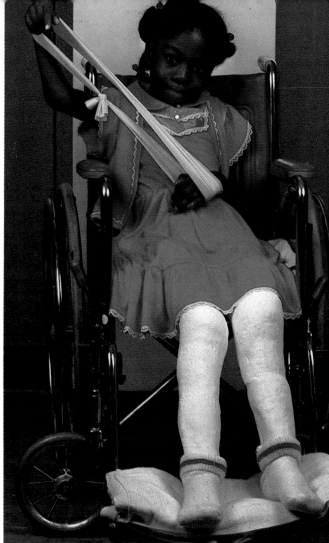

Nine-year-old Yolanda Oliver, a victim of juvenile rheumatoid arthritis, pulls and stretches a large rubber band to strengthen her arm muscles. The casts on Yolanda's legs help straighten them; her casts will be changed every few days for several weeks as surgeons manipulate her joints into alignment. When the casts are removed, she will have to learn to walk again.

Intense concentration on her face, Vera Drain reaches up to drop a plastic ring onto a tall wooden peg. The reaching increases her ability to move her shoulder and elbow joints, while the act of fitting the rings over the peg exercises her hands and fingers.

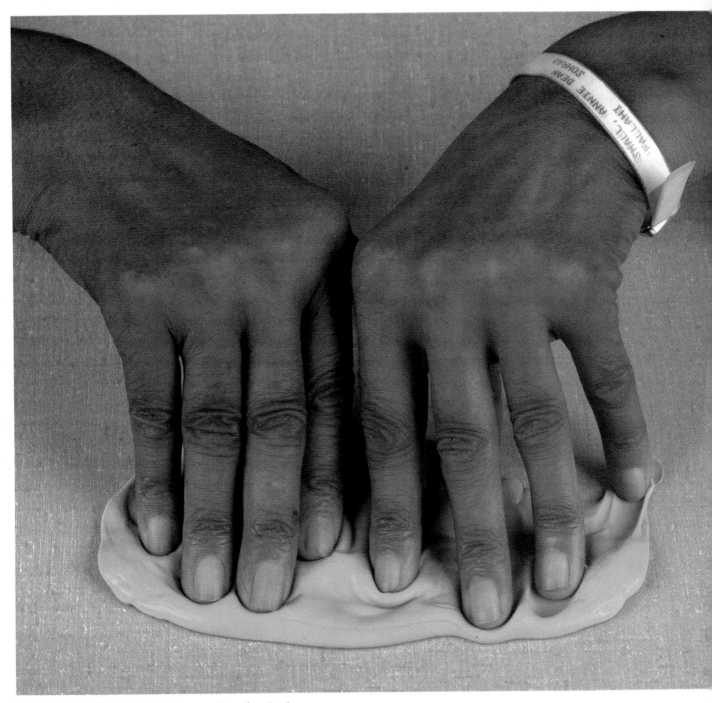

*Kneading malleable putty helps counteract loss of motion in
finger joints and loss of strength in muscles. The putty is available
in different degrees of stiffness, and the various consistencies
are marked by color; this green type is fairly stiff.*

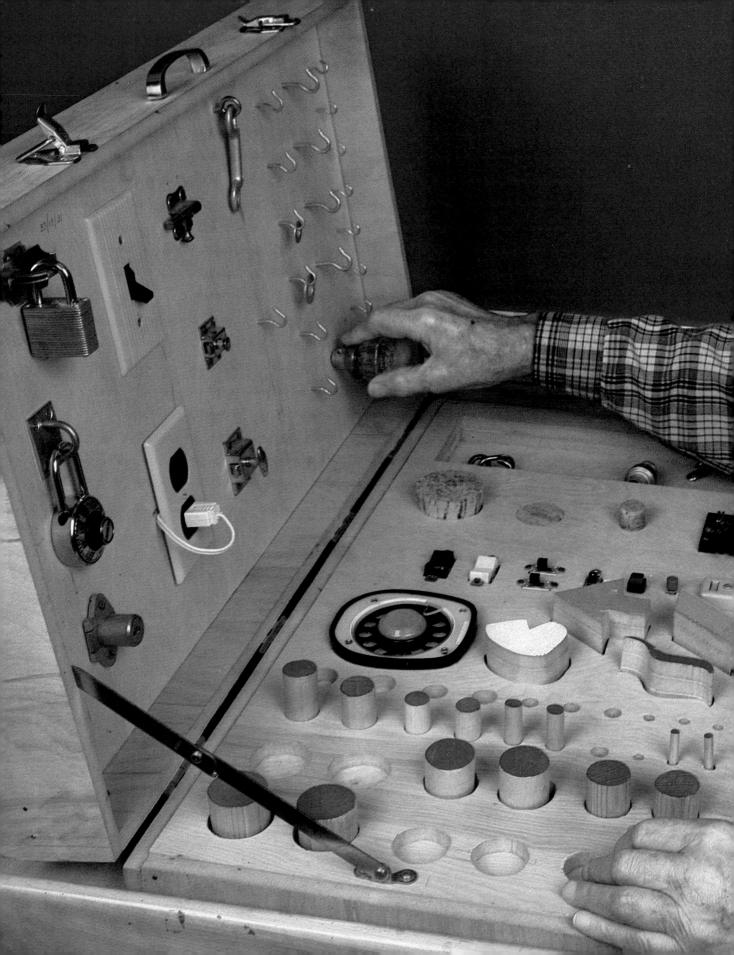

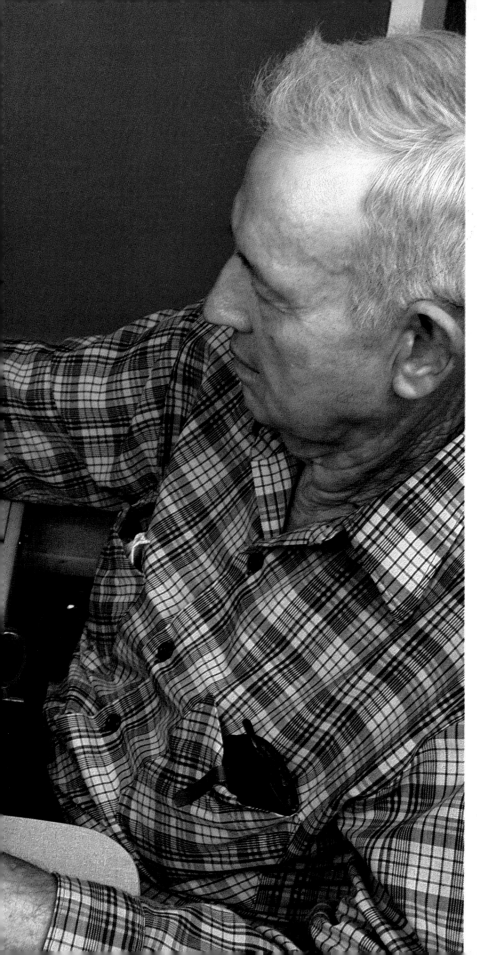

Omri Preston turns a doorknob, one of many household devices in a set specially assembled to provide practice in tasks routinely encountered at home and work— opening a combination lock, dialing a telephone, pushing a plug into a wall outlet. Other tasks offered by the device, such as forcing corks into small holes, help develop general strength and dexterity.

An encyclopedia of symptoms

The human body's ability to move—indeed, its ability to breathe and pump blood and, in that sense, to exist—is predicated on an amazing collection of bones, muscles, tendons and other tissues that must work in concert. If trouble strikes, it is important to know whether you should see a doctor immediately, whether you can wait, or whether you should treat yourself at home. Bones, muscles and nerves are all interconnected, and pain in one area may reflect a problem elsewhere. The most common disorders of the frame are described below, listed alphabetically by the symptoms that can be felt or seen. The condition that causes the symptom or group of symptoms appears in small capital letters.

ANKLE PAIN. The ankle is subject to almost all of the common ailments that affect joints, but particularly to FRACTURES, to SPRAINS and, at the back of the ankle where the Achilles' tendon joins the calf muscle to the heel, to TENDINITIS (see JOINT PAIN). It can also be the site of pains originating in the feet, such as MORTON'S FOOT or OVERPRONATION (see FOOT PAIN).

If severe ankle pain near the Achilles' tendon occurs with a sudden loss of foot movement, a RUPTURED TENDON may be indicated. Consult a physician immediately.

BACK PAIN. Back pain, acute or chronic, is perhaps the most common—and most difficult to diagnose—of all ailments affecting the frame. Some such pains arise from internal organs rather than the skeleton. Consult a physician if any back pain is severe, persistent or recurrent.

● **Back pain that occurs suddenly or without prior warning** can indicate any of several problems involving the frame.

If severe low-back pain occurs suddenly and with extreme tightness of the lower-back muscles, the cause may be an ACUTE LUMBOSACRAL STRAIN, a stretching or tearing of the muscles or ligaments that hold the spine together. When such pain strikes, lie down or have someone help you to bed. Lie on your back or side, not on your stomach, and remain in bed, except to go to the bathroom, until the pain lessens. Apply heat to relieve pain. Consult a physician if pain persists for more than two weeks, if there is pain radiating down the back of the leg, or if pain is accompanied by fever or weakness.

If acute low-back pain is accompanied by sudden pain in the back of the thigh, buttock or calf, and by numbness or tingling in the leg or foot, the cause may be a HERNIATED or RUPTURED INTERVERTEBRAL DISC, more commonly called a slipped disc. Consult a physician immediately. Absolute rest is essential.

If acute back pain occurs after a major injury, a FRACTURE or FRACTURE-DISLOCATION of the spine may be indicated. Consult a physician immediately.

If acute back pain occurs, with or without shooting leg pain, in an older individual, the cause may be a COMPRESSION FRACTURE, the collapsing of a spinal bone. This may be the result of OSTEOPOROSIS, or thinned bone. See a doctor if the pain is severe or persists after two weeks of bed rest and heat treatments.

● **Chronic back pain, as opposed to the acute variety,** can arise from structural disorders, ranging from simple poor posture to serious inherited conditions.

If chronic back pain is accompanied by extreme overweight, the cause may be excess STRAIN on the back and abdominal muscles. Consult a physician, who probably will prescribe weight loss and exercises for the back.

If chronic back pain occurs during pregnancy, the cause is probably excess STRAIN on the back muscles due to increased weight. Perform daily back-strengthening exercises *(pages 64-65),* use a firm mattress and avoid high-heeled shoes. Massage and local heat also may help reduce pain.

If chronic back pain occurs in an elderly individual and is associated with stiffness, particularly in the morning or after prolonged sitting, and if the pain is aggravated by cold, damp weather and relieved by rest and local heat, the cause may be OSTEOARTHRITIS of the spine, a degenerative disorder that affects the cartilage of the spinal bones. Consult a physician promptly if pain is severe.

If chronic back pain occurs in a person whose spine curves sideways, the problem may be SCOLIOSIS. The curvature usually first appears in childhood, with pain occurring years later. Consult a physician at the first signs of scoliosis.

If chronic back pain strikes the lower back of a young man and is associated with back stiffness, the cause may be ANKYLOSING SPONDYLITIS, an inflammatory disease of the spine. Ninety per cent of the cases occur in men, and although it normally begins in the lower back, it can later involve higher spinal areas. Consult a physician, but you can wait until the next day.

BONE PAIN. Bone pain can result from structural disorders, such as those that are caused by injury, as well as from VIRUSES and BACTERIAL INFECTIONS.

● **Severe pain after injury that is accompanied by swelling, tenderness and loss of function** can indicate a FRACTURE, a broken bone. Consult a physician immediately. Apply ice, and elevate and immobilize the affected area.

● **Localized bone pain associated with swelling, tenderness and fever** can indicate OSTEOMYELITIS, a bacterial infection of the bone. Consult a physician immediately.

● **Localized bone pain that is dull or aching and often is worse at night** may indicate a BONE TUMOR, an abnormal growth in the bone. Consult a physician promptly.

ELBOW PAIN.

The elbow is a frequent site of most of the acute and chronic pains that affect the joints. It is particularly prone to BURSITIS, an inflammation of a fluid-filled sac, or bursa, located along the joint, and to TENDINITIS—tennis elbow—an irritation of the tendon that connects forearm muscles to the arm bone (see JOINT PAIN). The most common types of elbow pain will generally disappear with rest.

If elbow pain persists, with swelling or reddening, a tendon may be torn. Consult a physician promptly.

FEVER.

Fever—the elevation of body temperature above the normal 98.6° F. (37° C.)—can be a sign of dozens of minor and major disorders. Only occasionally is it associated with specific bone and muscle problems.

● **Fever that is associated with a hot, painful, swollen joint** may indicate SEPTIC ARTHRITIS, a bacterial joint infection. Consult a physician immediately.

● **Fever that occurs with painful joints in a child or adolescent** who has suffered a sore throat within the previous two weeks may suggest RHEUMATIC FEVER, an inflammatory disease that affects the joints and the heart. Consult a physician immediately.

● **Fever that is accompanied by such chronic joint pains as painful, swollen fingers** may indicate RHEUMATOID ARTHRITIS, a chronic inflammatory disease of the joints. Consult a physician within several days.

FINGER PAIN. The fingers are prone to many of the ills and injuries that affect joints—and especially to SPRAINS, DISLOCATIONS, RHEUMATOID ARTHRITIS, OSTEOARTHRITIS, and SEPTIC ARTHRITIS (see JOINT PAIN). Delicate and vulnerable, the fingers are also subject to FRACTURES (see BONE PAIN).

FOOT PAIN. Pains in the feet can result from conditions ranging from simple fatigue to serious structural defects; their origins can be internal, as when a bone breaks, or external, as when a skin eruption such as ATHLETE'S FOOT occurs. Foot pain can affect the entire foot, or it can strike one of its parts (see TOE PAIN, HEEL PAIN). And it can, when accompanied by thickened toenails and cold or bluish skin, indicate blood-flow disorders, usually brought on by ARTERIOSCLEROSIS, hardening of the arteries; or by DIABETES, an abnormality of the body's sugar-processing system.

● **Pain that is confined to the ball of the foot** may suggest any of several ailments.

If pain in the ball of the foot is felt as a burning sensation and gets worse when the foot bears weight, the cause may be METATARSALGIA, a tissue inflammation that primarily affects women who wear shoes with high heels and pointed toes. Thick, toughened skin—CALLUSES—on the ball of the foot can increase the pain. To reduce pain, wear low-heeled, roomy shoes. Consult a foot doctor if pain is persistent.

If pain at the ball of the foot is localized near the junction with the second toe, you should examine your feet to see if your big toe is shorter than your second toe. Many people's second toes are their longest; that fact generally is of no significance unless accompanied by foot or knee pain. The painful condition is called MORTON'S FOOT; if you suspect that you have it, consult a foot doctor.

If pain at the ball of the foot is confined to the area between the third and fourth toes, and if the pain radiates forward into the toes, the cause may be a MORTON'S NEUROMA, a thickened nerve caught between the two bones. Pain may be worse when the foot bears weight; it may be relieved by roomier shoes. Consult a foot doctor if pain is severe or persistent.

● **Pain in the entire foot** may indicate a structural problem.

If pain is felt throughout the foot but primarily under the arch, the cause may be excessive PRONATION, a turning-in of the foot and ankle that produces a flattened arch. Sometimes called FLAT FEET or FALLEN ARCHES, this condition can produce an unnatural gait and frequently causes pain in the ankle, knee, leg and back. (Feet that merely appear flat need cause no concern; only when painful turning-in occurs need you be alarmed.) Consult a foot doctor if such pain persists.

If pain is generalized along the bottom of the foot and increases on weight-bearing, the cause may be a STRESS FRACTURE, a small crack in a foot bone. This usually happens to people who do a great deal of walking, marching or running. Rest usually results in complete healing, but see a doctor if pain persists for more than a week.

● **Pain confined to the skin of the foot** can be caused by such common toe problems as CALLUSES and CORNS (see TOE PAIN). Or it may have other origins.

If skin pain is localized to a small cauliflower-like growth on the bottom of the foot, the cause may be a PLANTAR WART, a viral infection of the skin. The growth can be removed by a doctor if pain is annoying.

HEEL PAIN.

Heels are subject to many painful conditions—including the common joint ailment BURSITIS (see JOINT PAIN) and certain special variations of that affliction.

● **Heel pain that is confined to the bottom of the heel** may be due to PLANTAR BURSITIS, an inflammation of the cushiony bursal sacs on the underside of the heel. To reduce pain, wear cushioned shoes or insert a doughnut-shaped pad under the sore area.

● **Heel pain that is confined to the back of the heel** may be caused by ACHILLES' TENDON BURSITIS, inflammation of the cushiony sacs, or bursae, that pad the Achilles' tendon. The ailment often is due to friction of the shoe on the skin. Wear low-heeled shoes that fit properly *(page 75)*. If pain persists, see a doctor.

● **Heel pain at the bottom of the heel that spreads out along the foot** can indicate PLANTAR FASCITIS, a stretching or tearing of the connective tissue, or fascia, at the bottom of the foot. Mild pain can be treated by rest and local heat—try soaking your feet in hot water. Massage the bottom of the foot and wear flexible shoes with a good heel cushion. If pain persists after two weeks, see a doctor.

HIP PAIN. Because the hip is a large, weight-bearing joint, it is especially prone to the ills that afflict joints—particularly OSTEOARTHRITIS and BURSITIS (see JOINT PAIN). Hip pain can also result from problems with the feet, such as MORTON'S FOOT, OVERPRONATION and STRESS FRACTURE (see FOOT PAIN), or from back trouble (see BACK PAIN) and knee disorders (see KNEE PAIN). Certain hip pains are very common and important.

● **If hip pain is severe and motion is limited,** the cause may be a FRACTURED FEMUR, a broken thighbone. Consult a physician immediately. This fairly common occurrence usually affects older individuals—particularly elderly women—and can be due to OSTEOPOROSIS, or thinned bone. It can strike after an injury, such as a fall, or seemingly without cause.

JAW PAIN. Jaw pain usually is due to dental problems, but it can suggest many ills, including ANGINA PECTORIS—a gripping, seizing pain in the chest, jaw or arm, or all three, that signals insufficient blood flow to the heart. Contact a doctor immediately.

● **Jaw pain that is accompanied by a snapping or popping sound or feeling** just in front of either ear may indicate a TEMPOROMANDIBULAR JOINT SUBLUXATION, a partial separation of the jaw joint. There may be locking or stiffness of the joint. Consult a physician if pain persists or if locking is recurrent.

JOINT PAIN. Pain in the joints is an extremely common complaint, affecting people of all ages. It usually originates in the bones, muscles and connective tissues of the frame, but not always. Joint pain can signal VIRAL INFECTION, INFLUENZA and SICKLE-CELL ANEMIA, a hereditary disease of the red blood cells in black children. It also can suggest RHEUMATIC FEVER, an inflammatory

disease that normally affects children and can severely damage the heart. In that ailment, joint pain usually is preceded by a sore throat and is accompanied by severe joint swelling and tenderness, skin rash or lumps under the skin, unusual muscle movements or chest pain, and difficult breathing. Consult a physician immediately.

● **Joint pain that occurs after injury** may indicate one of several ailments affecting the frame.

If joint pain occurs immediately after a twisting injury, it usually indicates a SPRAIN, a stretching or tearing of the ligaments that hold the joint together. The injury normally causes sharp pain at first, then after a few hours an aching pain accompanied by swelling, tenderness and restricted movement. Apply ice, elevate the joint and keep weight off it until the worst pain passes—usually two days or so. Have the sprain evaluated by a doctor within a few days.

If severe joint pain develops immediately after injury and is associated with loss of joint function, a DISLOCATION or FRACTURE may be indicated. The joint may appear deformed. Obtain medical treatment immediately. Pain is usually severe, unremitting and unresponsive to conventional first aid, such as that for SPRAINS.

● **Joint pain can be localized and characterized by occasional or recurrent acute attacks.**

If localized joint pain is sudden and occurs on joint movement, and if it is associated with swelling or a knob under the skin near the joint, the cause may be BURSITIS, an inflammation of the fluid-filled sacs called bursae that lubricate most joints. Attacks may follow injury or overuse of the joint. Consult a physician if pain does not subside after three to four days or if attacks recur frequently. Meanwhile, rest the affected joint, apply ice packs or cold compresses during the first 24 hours, and moist heat thereafter. Take aspirin.

If localized joint pain occurs suddenly, is severe and is accompanied by swelling, redness and tenderness, GOUT, a blood abnormality, may be suggested. Such pain often affects the big toe of men. Consult a physician as soon as possible.

If localized joint pain is mild to moderate and occurs a day or so after strenuous activity, the cause may be TENDINITIS, an inflammation of the tissue that attaches muscles to bone. Pain is usually worse in the morning and may abate if activity is reduced. Avoid strenuous exercise until pain is gone. Gentle stretching exercises, followed after several days by more active exercises to strengthen the muscles of the affected area, will help prevent recurrence.

● **Joint pains—either localized or generalized—that prove chronic rather than acute** may indicate a potentially crippling or disabling condition.

If chronic joint pain is dull or aching and the affected joints are swollen and are stiffer in the morning than later in the day, or if the pain occurs with fever, weakness or weight loss, the cause may be RHEUMATOID ARTHRITIS, an inflammatory disease of the synovium, the inner lining of joints. The fingers and wrists are frequent sites of such pain. Nodules or lumps under the skin may be found, most commonly on the forearm. Consult a physician immediately if symptoms are severe, within several days if they are not.

If chronic joint pain affects an older person and is made worse by movement but is relieved by rest, the cause may be OSTEO-ARTHRITIS or DEGENERATIVE JOINT DISEASE, a wearing and rough-ening of the smooth cartilage cap on the ends of bones. The fingers, back, hip and knee are the most frequent sites. Such pain may be accompanied by temporary stiffness after rest or inactivity; it is seldom accompanied by fever, weakness or weight loss—signs of the less common RHEUMATOID ARTHRITIS. See a doctor if pain is severe or persistent. Avoid weight-bearing and overuse of the af-fected joints; apply heat and take aspirin for temporary pain relief.

● **Joint pain in children or adolescents** may indicate disorders not generally seen in adults. Except for the minor temporary joint aches associated with colds or flu, all joint pain in children should be evaluated by a physician.

If joint pain occurs suddenly in a child and is severe enough so that the child is reluctant to move the joint, and if it is accompanied by local heat, swelling, tenderness and such signs of infection as fever and ill appearance, the cause may be SEPTIC ARTHRITIS, a bacterial infection of the joint. Consult a physician immediately.

If a child develops joint pain that is associated with high fever, skin rash, chest or eye pain, the cause may be JUVENILE RHEUMA-TOID ARTHRITIS, a chronic inflammatory disease of the joint lining, or synovium. Consult a physician as soon as possible.

KNEE PAIN.

The knee is a common site for a host of such joint ailments and injuries as SPRAINS, BURSITIS and OSTEOARTHRITIS (see JOINT PAIN). The knee also is subject to ailments all its own.

● **Knee pain that occurs with locking of the joint**—inability to bend the knee—may indicate an injury or the presence of a ''loose body,'' a small bit of detached tissue inside the joint. The particles, or ''joint mice,'' occasionally produce a clicking sound when the knee is bent. Consult a physician if pain persists.

● **Knee pain in young adults that occurs near the kneecap** and is aggravated by bending the knee or climbing stairs may indicate CHONDROMALACIA PATELLA, or softening of the cartilage of the kneecap. Such pain may be accompanied by a grating sensation on movement. Consult a physician within several days.

● **Knee pain that is felt in and around the front of the knee and that is made worse by exercise** is commonly called RUNNER'S KNEE. The term is somewhat misleading, for the pain usually is caused by an abnormality of the foot such as MORTON'S FOOT or OVERPRONATION (see FOOT PAIN). To treat runner's knee you must correct the foot ailment. A good pair of sturdy running shoes with arch supports usually will suffice.

LEG PAIN.

Most leg pains result from relatively minor muscle problems (see MUSCLE PAIN). Yet they can signal potentially serious blood-vessel disorders, such as INTERMITTENT CLAUDICATION, in which hardened tissues restrict blood flow to the legs, and THROMBOPHLEBITIS, in which clots form in leg veins. Consult a physician promptly if leg pain is accompanied by skin changes such as smooth, shiny skin with hair loss, bluish-red discoloration or skin ulcers. The feet may feel cool to the touch and the toenails may be thickened.

● **Leg pain that occurs with back pain** may indicate SCIATICA, compression of the large sciatic nerve near the spine. The pain normally is felt first in the buttocks or hip, then radiates down the back of the leg to the calf and sometimes into the foot. Numbness, tingling or weakness may be present. Consult a physician promptly.

● **Leg pain that is felt in the front of the lower leg**—along the shin—can be due to SHIN SPLINTS, pulled shin muscles. Rest, ele-vate your feet and shins and apply ice. Consult a physician if pain persists for more than three weeks.

MUSCLE PAIN.

Muscle aches or pains are extremely com-mon and can have causes ranging from simple bumps and bruises to overexercising, INFLUENZA and VIRAL INFECTIONS. Minor aches and pains can be treated at home—rest, apply heat and take aspirin. For severe pain that is persistent or that is associated with loss of function, consult a physician immediately.

● **Muscle pain that occurs during or after exercise** can have several causes.

If localized severe muscle pain occurs suddenly during exer-cise, a MUSCLE STRAIN, or a ''pulled muscle,'' may be the cause. In this condition, muscle fibers are overstretched or torn and can heal only if given adequate rest. The most common sites are the ham-string muscle on the back of the thigh, and the muscles of the groin and shoulder. Consult a physician immediately if pain is severe or if it is accompanied by loss of function in the affected area. For home treatment, apply ice to the injury, but use ice for only one day or less. On the day after injury, apply heat—from an electric heating pad or a towel soaked in hot water. Rest until the pain is nearly gone—this may take two to 14 days—and then begin gentle exer-cises, building up gradually to your previous exercise level.

If localized severe muscle pain occurs with a knotted feeling during or after exercise, a MUSCLE CRAMP, an extreme muscle con-traction, may be indicated. The muscle usually will relax by itself within several minutes. To hasten that process, gently massage or squeeze the cramped muscle and stretch it at the same time.

If muscles become painful and cramped during exercise in hot weather, the cause may be HEAT CRAMPS, the result of a chemical imbalance produced when large amounts of salt and potassium are sweated out through the skin. Obtain medical treatment promptly if cramps are severe or do not relax within a few minutes. Otherwise, drink water and add more fruit and vegetables to your diet.

If a sudden pain in the side occurs during exercise, it may indicate a DIAPHRAGMATIC SPASM, a "stitch" or pain in the muscle that controls breathing. Other possible causes include gas in the colon and eating just before exercise. Slow down or rest and the pain will subside within a few minutes.

MUSCLE WEAKNESS. Muscle weakness that is mild and generalized may be a sign of fatigue or infection. See a doctor if symptoms persist for more than a week. Persistent muscle weakness that is mild at first, then worsens, may signal a more serious condition.
● **Progressive muscle weakness** can indicate disease of the muscles or nerves, or both.

If progressive muscle weakness occurs in a child or adolescent and is associated with enlarged but soft calf or forearm muscles, the cause may be MUSCULAR DYSTROPHY, a hereditary and degenerative muscle disorder that can lead to loss of muscle function. Consult a physician promptly.

If progressive muscle weakness occurs in a young adult and is associated with easy and excessive fatigue of face, eye, jaw or mouth muscles, the cause may be MYASTHENIA GRAVIS, a disorder of the chemical connection between nerves and muscles. Consult a physician immediately. Because the muscle fatigue associated with this disorder increases with activity, symptoms may worsen toward the end of the day.

If progressive muscle weakness occurs in a middle-aged adult and is associated with wasting of the limbs, the cause may be AMYOTROPHIC LATERAL SCLEROSIS, a disorder in which the nerves of the spinal cord and brain deteriorate. (The disorder is also called LOU GEHRIG'S DISEASE.) Muscles may be hyperactive or spastic as well as weak. Consult a physician promptly.

NECK PAIN. Most neck pains are minor, if annoying. Some are associated with TENSION HEADACHES; others are more appropriately considered disorders of the upper part of the back, or the cervical spine. Such common back ailments as DEGENERATIVE DISC DISEASE and HERNIATED INTRAVERTEBRAL DISCS can strike the neck, as can such back injuries as FRACTURES and DISLOCATIONS (see BACK PAIN). The neck also can fall prey to a host of muscle and joint ailments, particularly MUSCLE SPASM (see MUSCLE PAIN) and OSTEOARTHRITIS (see JOINT PAIN). Yet the neck is known for one type of pain all its own.

If neck pain occurs several hours after an injury in which the head is snapped violently forward or backward, such as the "whiplash" of an automobile accident, the cause may be an ACUTE CERVICAL STRAIN, a stretching of the muscles and ligaments that support the bones of the neck. Consult a physician as soon as possible. Pain may be accompanied by restricted neck motion, headache, dizziness, nausea, loss of balance and blurred vision.

NECK STIFFNESS. A stiff neck is an extremely common complaint; usually it is produced by a MUSCLE SPASM (see MUSCLE PAIN). Sometimes it can arise from problems that affect the cervical or neck joints, such as OSTEOARTHRITIS (see JOINT PAIN). Rarely does it suggest a truly serious disorder. Consult a physician immediately, however, if a stiff neck is accompanied by severe, unremitting headache, or by nausea and vomiting, skin rash, behavior changes or loss of consciousness.

If a stiff neck occurs in an infant and the neck is twisted to one side, TORTICOLLIS, or "WRY NECK," may be the cause. The ailment may be congenital or may be acquired after an injury or infection. Consult a physician within several days.

SHOULDER PAIN. The shoulder is a common site of the ills and injuries that can affect most joints, including TENDINITIS and BURSITIS (see JOINT PAIN). It is also stricken by ailments unique to it, and by pains arising in such internal organs as the heart, lungs, liver and gall bladder. Consult a physician immediately if shoulder pain is limited to the right arm or to the back of the shoulder, or if it is accompanied by chest pain, pain in the jaw, sweating, nausea or vomiting—possible signs of serious internal ailments.
● **Acute shoulder pain that develops after a sudden injury or strenuous work,** or that is associated with an inability to lift the arm away from the chest, may indicate a ROTATOR-CUFF TEAR, a tear of the muscle or tendons surrounding the shoulder joint. Consult a physician immediately.
● **Shoulder pain that occurs with tenderness at the front or side of the shoulder** and is associated with restricted motion may indicate CALCIFIC TENDINITIS, a common condition in which bits of calcium are deposited in the tissues around the joint. Initial attacks may be sudden and severe, followed by a dull ache that characterizes the chronic phase. Consult a physician within a day or so.
● **Chronic shoulder pain that is dull and aching,** and that occurs with progressive limitation of movement may indicate ADHESIVE CAPSULITIS, or "frozen shoulder," a condition in which the tis-

sues surrounding the joint become stiff and tight. Consult a physician promptly.

SWELLING. Swelling, also called EDEMA, can be a sign of many ailments affecting the bones, muscles and connective tissues, but it also can have other—and occasionally extremely serious—origins. If you press on a swollen area and your fingers sink in and leave a depression, or pit, the cause may be a serious internal disorder such as KIDNEY DISEASE, LIVER DISEASE, or HEART FAILURE. Consult a physician immediately. Swelling that is not of the ''pitting'' variety can be an indication of an INSECT BITE or of an ALLERGIC REACTION. Such swelling usually is confined to small patches and is accompanied by itching or reddened skin.

● **Swelling that is localized and that is not of the pitting variety** may indicate a SPRAIN, TENDINITIS, BURSITIS, or any of several joint injuries and ills (see JOINT PAIN). To reduce swelling and pain, apply ice, and elevate and rest the affected area. Consult a physician if swelling persists after a week of home treatment.

TOE PAIN. Many painful toe conditions result from wearing shoes that are too tight and narrow; the treatment is simply shoes that fit properly. Toes also are subject to ailments and injuries that affect bones, such as FRACTURES (see BONE PAIN), and joints, such as SPRAINS and OSTEOARTHRITIS (see JOINT PAIN). Severe or recurrent toe pain, however, can suggest conditions that require immediate medical treatment. These include FROSTBITE and GOUT, a blood abnormality marked by severe pain, swelling, tenderness and restricted motion in the big toe, mainly in men.

● **Toe pain often is the result of abnormalities of the skin.**

If pain is localized to an area where the skin rubs against the shoe, the probable cause is a HARD CORN, a thickening of the skin caused by irritation. Do not attempt to remove or cut a corn yourself. Temporary relief may be obtained by placing a doughnut-shaped pad over the sore area. Correct shoe fit is mandatory.

If pain is confined to an area between the toes and is not associated with itching, the cause may be a SOFT CORN, a moist thickening of the skin caused by two toes pressing on each other, most commonly because of tight shoes. Place some cotton between the toes to separate them and reduce the friction.

If pain and itching occur between the toes, or if there is scaling of the skin of the toes or soles, the cause is most likely a fungus infection such as ATHLETE'S FOOT. Keep your feet clean and dry and apply fungicide containing micronazole nitrate, undecylenic acid or tolnaftate, available at drugstores.

● **Painful toes can be the result of conditions affecting the nails.**

If pain occurs along the edge of the nail of the big toe, the probable cause is an INGROWN TOENAIL, in which the nail grows down and into the skin. This can be caused by tight shoes or by improper nail-cutting *(page 70).* Mild cases may be treated by tucking a small piece of cotton under the corner of the nail to raise it away from the skin. Consult a foot doctor promptly if the skin becomes infected—red, hot, swollen and tender.

If a toenail becomes black but is not painful, and if you are in the habit of jogging or walking for exercise, the cause may be RUNNER'S TOE, a generally harmless condition that primarily affects runners whose toes get jammed into the ends of their shoes. The nail may fall off after a few weeks; it will grow back in about two months. Consult a foot doctor if pain develops or if the blackened nail remains in place for longer than one to two months.

● **Painful toes that have unusual shapes or a deformed appearance** may suggest any of several conditions.

If the big toe is crooked and points inward toward the second toe, and if there is pain along the outer edge of the big toe, the cause may be a BUNION, also called HALLUX VALGUS, an enlargement of the bone and a twisting of the toe. The bunion itself may be painless, but constant friction between the skin and the shoe can cause irritation and pain. Wearing a wide shoe may provide enough room to prevent friction and reduce pain. A sore spot can also be covered with a doughnut-shaped pad.

If a toe is painful and crooked, with its tip pointing down excessively, the cause may be a HAMMERTOE DEFORMITY, in which the toe joints become locked in this abnormal position. The second toe is most commonly affected. This condition may be painless and nothing to worry about, but painful CORNS or CALLUSES—deposits of tough, encrusted skin—can form on either the top or bottom of the toe where the skin rubs against the shoe. Wearing shoes with enough toe room or placing a doughnut-shaped pad over the sore area often will reduce the pain.

WRIST PAIN. The wrist is a frequent site of injury and is prone to most of the ailments that affect joints generally, and particularly to SPRAINS (see JOINT PAIN). But there are several maladies that affect the wrist exclusively and require professional attention if pain persists.

● **Dull, aching pain associated with a firm nodule or bump under the skin** may indicate a GANGLION CYST, a small swelling of the tissue near the wrist; it is usually filled with a thick fluid. In some cases, nodules appear without pain.

● **Pain, burning or tingling along the wrist, forearm or hand** that is made worse by bending the wrist at a sharp angle may indicate CARPAL TUNNEL SYNDROME, a condition that results from the compression of a nerve as it crosses the wrist.

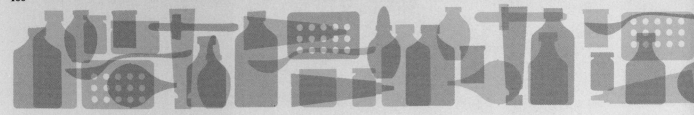

Drugs for an aching body

Drugs to relieve body aches are almost as numerous as the ailments that cause them. Most are painkillers, but many do more than relieve pain; they attack its source. Aspirin, for example, lessens joint and muscle pain by controlling inflammation.

In this table—prepared by Christopher S. Conner, Director of the Rocky Mountain Drug Consultation Center—the drugs most commonly used are listed by generic names, with trade names appearing below each entry. Drugs containing more than one active ingredient are starred; prescription drugs are marked Rx.

Heed these basic precautions: Pregnant women should consult a physician before taking any drug. Anyone taking a drug that causes drowsiness should avoid alcohol or other depressants, and should not drive. Consult a physician if serious side effects appear: Sore throat, unusual bruising or bleeding, or weakness may indicate a reduced blood-cell count; yellowing of skin or whites of the eyes suggests liver damage.

DRUG	Intended effect	Minor side effects	Serious side effects	Special cautions
ACETAMINOPHEN **TYLENOL** **NEBS** **DATRIL**	Relieves mild to moderate pain in muscles and joints	Dizziness; diarrhea, upset stomach	Liver damage or hepatitis; reduced blood-cell counts	Consult doctor before taking if you have liver disease.
ALLOPURINOL (Rx) **ZYLOPRIM**	Prevents gout	Diarrhea; nausea; drowsiness; stomach pain	Skin rash; liver damage; kidney damage; kidney stones; reduced blood-cell counts; inflammation of nerves	Consult doctor before taking if you have kidney or liver disease. Drink 8 to 10 glasses of water a day while taking this drug. Inform doctor of tingling or numbness of hands or feet. Effects may be reduced by alcohol and diuretics, drugs that eliminate fluid. Effects of warfarin, a blood-thinner, may be increased by this drug.
ASPIRIN **ASCRIPTIN** **BUFFERIN** **CAMA** **ECOTRIN** **MEASURIN**	Relieves pain and inflammation	Upset stomach; ringing in the ears	Bleeding and erosion of the stomach lining (ulcers); hearing loss; allergic reactions, such as tightness in chest or wheezing; slowed blood clotting; liver damage	Consult doctor before taking if you have peptic ulcer, liver disease, bleeding disorders, or a history of allergies or asthma. Do not exceed more than 10 tablets (50 grains) in 24 hours. Do not take tablets that smell like vinegar—odor indicates presence of acetic acid, a by-product of decomposition that can irritate mouth or stomach. Take with full glass of milk or water to lessen stomach irritation. Stop taking 1 week before any surgery.
CARISOPRODOL (Rx) **SOMA** **RELA** **SOMA COMPOUND***	Relieves muscle spasm and its pain	Drowsiness; nausea; nervousness; headache	Severe dizziness or fainting; allergic reactions, such as skin rash, difficulty breathing, itching; depression; extreme weakness; confusion; temporary loss of limb control or vision	Consult doctor before taking if you have been diagnosed as having porphyria, a disorder of metabolism, or if you are allergic to meprobamate, a tranquilizer, or carbromal, a sedative.
CHLOROQUINE (Rx) **ARALEN**	Relieves symptoms of rheumatoid arthritis	Nausea; diarrhea; abdominal cramps; skin rash; headache	Damage to the retina and cornea; reduced blood-cell counts; muscle weakness; ringing in ears; mental or behavioral changes	Consult doctor before taking if you have blood disorders, liver disease, eye disturbances involving the retina, or mental illness. Take with milk to lessen stomach upset. Inform doctor of blurred or reduced vision—signs of eye damage.

* Combination drug. Refer also to other active ingredients on label.

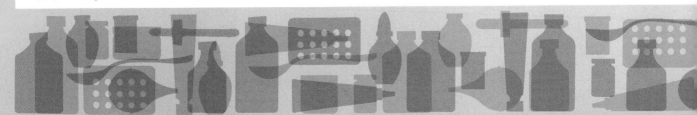

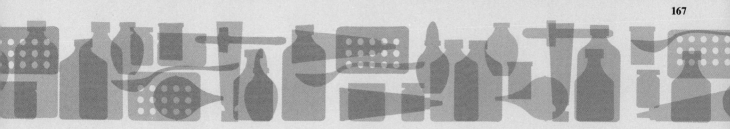

DRUG	Intended effect	Minor side effects	Serious side effects	Special cautions
CHLORPHENESIN CARBAMATE (Rx) MAOLATE	Relieves muscle spasm and its pain	Drowsiness; dizziness; upset stomach; nervousness; headache	Skin rash; reduced blood-cell counts	Consult doctor before taking if you are breast feeding; this drug is excreted in breast milk and may cause sedation in the infant.
CHLORZOXAZONE (Rx) PARAFLEX PARAFON FORTE*	Relieves muscle spasm and its pain	Drowsiness; dizziness; nausea; vomiting; headache	Bleeding from stomach; allergic reactions, such as skin rash and itching; reduced blood-cell counts; liver damage	Consult doctor before taking if you have liver disease. Inform doctor of bloody or black, tarry stools—signs of stomach bleeding.
CHOLINE MAGNESIUM TRISALICYLATE (Rx) TRILISATE	Relieves mild to moderate pain and inflammation, principally in arthritis	Indigestion; ringing in ears	Severe nausea or vomiting; stomach bleeding; creation or activation of ulcers; hearing loss; allergic reactions, such as tightness in the chest or wheezing	Consult doctor before taking if you have a peptic ulcer. Take with a full glass of milk or water to lessen stomach upset. Notify doctor of persistent ringing in ears, headache or dizziness—signs of overdose. Risk of ulcers is increased if taken with other anti-inflammation drugs or with alcohol. Notify doctor of black, tarry stools—signs of stomach bleeding.
CHOLINE SALICYLATE ARTHROPAN LIQUID	All effects similar to CHOLINE MAGNESIUM TRISALICYLATE			
CODEINE (Rx) TYLENOL WITH CODEINE* EMPIRIN WITH CODEINE*	Relieves mild to moderate pain	Constipation; loss of appetite; upset stomach; drowsiness; dizziness; skin rash	Difficulty breathing; slow heart rate; fainting; liver damage	Consult doctor before taking if you have liver, respiratory or heart disease, or if you are pregnant. Drug dependence may occur with extended use.
COLCHICINE (Rx) COLCHICINE TABLETS COLBENEMID*	Relieves pain and inflammation in acute gout attacks	Nausea; vomiting; abdominal pain or diarrhea	Skin rash; reduced blood-cell counts; nerve inflammation; colon inflammation	Consult doctor before taking if you have heart, liver or kidney disease or stomach and intestinal disorders. Inform doctor of tingling or numbness of hands or feet—signs of nerve inflammation.
CORTISOL (Rx) CORTEF HYDROCORTONE	Relieves inflammation, principally in arthritis	Nausea; indigestion; menstrual irregularities; weight gain; insomnia; nervousness	Mental and emotional disturbances; potassium loss; bone disease; peptic ulcer; increased glucose levels in blood (diabetes); inflammation of the pancreas; increased pressure inside the eye (glaucoma); high blood pressure; muscle cramps or weakness; impaired immune response	Consult doctor before taking if you are taking digoxin or digitoxin, drugs that control heartbeat—may increase risk of irregular heartbeat. Consult doctor before taking if you have heart disease, diabetes mellitus, fungus infections, peptic ulcer or tuberculosis. Adhere to a low-salt diet as outlined by your doctor. Inform doctor of black, tarry stools—signs of stomach bleeding. Inform doctor of persistent muscle cramps or unusual tiredness—signs of potassium loss. Do not discontinue abruptly after prolonged use—withdrawal reactions may occur, such as fever, weakness, and dangerous decreases in blood pressure. Do not submit to any vaccinations or skin tests without consulting your doctor. Risk of ulcers is increased if drug is taken with other anti-inflammation drugs or with alcohol or aspirin. May interfere with effects of warfarin, a blood thinner, and drugs used to treat diabetes.

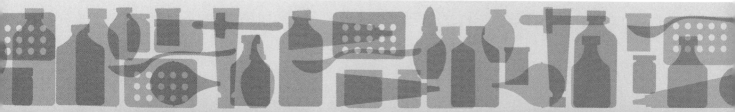

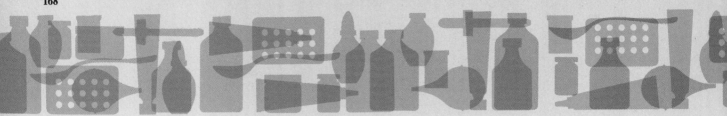

DRUG	Intended effect	Minor side effects	Serious side effects	Special cautions

CORTISONE (Rx)
  CORTONE
  CORTISONE
    ACETATE
    TABLETS
	All effects similar to CORTISOL			

CYCLOBENZAPRINE (Rx) **FLEXERIL**	Relieves muscle spasm and its pain	Drowsiness; dry mouth; dizziness; weakness; blurred vision; insomnia; rapid heart rate	Confusion, depression or hallucinations; difficulty breathing; difficulty urinating; allergic reactions such as skin rash or itching	Consult doctor before taking if you have heart disease or urination difficulties. Can cause severe reactions if taken with monoamine oxidase (MAO) inhibitors used to treat depression.

DEXAMETHASONE (Rx)
  DECADRON
  HEXADROL
  DEXONE TM
	All effects similar to CORTISOL			

DIAZEPAM (Rx) **VALIUM**	Relieves muscle spasm and its pain	Drowsiness; slurred speech; weakness; clumsiness	Depression; excited or agitated behavior; confusion; liver damage; reduced blood-cell counts; difficulty breathing	Drug dependence can occur with extended use, even at recommended doses. Consult doctor before taking if you have lung disease. Consult doctor before discontinuing after extended use; withdrawal symptoms can occur, including agitation, confusion and seizures. The effects of this drug are enhanced when taken with cimetidine, used for ulcers.
DIHYDROCODEINE BITARTRATE (Rx) **SYNALGOS-DC***	Relieves moderate to severe pain	Drowsiness; constipation; dizziness; upset stomach	Shortness of breath; slow heart rate	Consult doctor before taking if you have liver, heart or respiratory disease. Consult doctor before taking if you are pregnant—this drug can depress vital functions in the newborn. Drug dependence may result with extended use.
FENOPROFEN (Rx) **NALFON**	Relieves pain and inflammation	Drowsiness; nausea; diarrhea; dizziness; constipation; headache; stomach discomfort	Creation or activation of stomach ulcer; ringing in the ears; impaired vision; severe skin rash; fluid retention; decreased blood-cell counts; kidney damage	Consult doctor before taking if you have ulcers or have had unusual reactions to aspirin or other anti-inflammation drugs. Take with food or milk to lessen stomach upset. Risk of ulcers is increased if taken with other anti-inflammation drugs or with alcohol or aspirin. Notify doctor of black, tarry stools—signs of stomach bleeding. Notify doctor of swelling of legs or feet—signs of excess fluid retention. Notify doctor of painful urination or blood in the urine—signs of kidney damage.

HYDROCORTISONE (Rx)
  CORTEF
  HYDROCORTONE
	All effects similar to CORTISOL			

HYDROMORPHONE (Rx) **DILAUDID**	Relieves severe pain	Constipation; dizziness; drowsiness; nausea; vomiting; appetite loss	Difficulty breathing; slow heart rate; fainting	Consult doctor before taking if you have respiratory, liver or heart disease. Consult doctor before taking if you are pregnant—this drug can depress vital functions in the newborn.

* Combination drug. Refer also to other active ingredients on label.

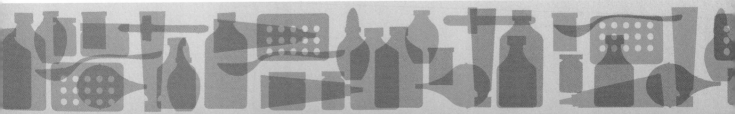

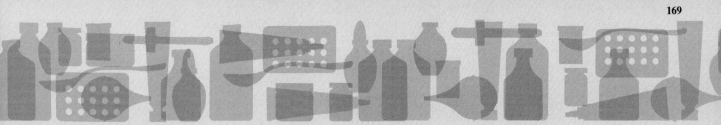

DRUG	Intended effect	Minor side effects	Serious side effects	Special cautions
HYDROXYCHLOR-OQUINE (Rx) **PLAQUENIL**	All effects similar to CHLOROQUINE			
IBUPROFEN (Rx) **MOTRIN**	All effects similar to FENOPROFEN			
INDOMETHACIN (Rx) **INDOCIN**	Relieves pain and inflammation, principally in arthritis	Headache; nausea; vomiting; dizziness	Stomach ulcers and bleeding; ringing in the ears; eye damage with prolonged use; fluid retention; liver damage; reduced blood-cell counts	Consult doctor before taking if you have liver disease, ulcers or other stomach problems. Take with food or milk to decrease the likelihood of stomach upset. Ulcers are more likely to occur if this drug is used with other anti-inflammation drugs, such as aspirin, or with alcohol. Increased likelihood of stomach bleeding if taken with warfarin, a blood-thinning drug. Notify doctor of blurred vision during prolonged use—signs of eye damage. Notify doctor of black, tarry stools—signs of stomach bleeding.
MAGNESIUM SALICYLATE (Rx) **MAGAN** **MOBIDIN** **TRIACT**	All effects similar to CHOLINE MAGNESIUM TRISALICYLATE			
MEPERIDINE (Rx) **DEMEROL**	Relieves moderate to severe pain	Constipation; dizziness; drowsiness; nausea; vomiting; appetite loss	Difficulty breathing; slow heart rate; fainting	Consult doctor before taking if you have respiratory, liver or heart disease. Consult doctor before taking if you are pregnant—this drug can depress vital functions in the newborn. Can cause severe reactions if taken with monoamine oxidase (MAO) inhibitors used to treat depression. Take judiciously: Dependence may result with extended use.
MEPROBAMATE (Rx) **EQUAGESIC***	Relieves anxiety that occasionally accompanies pain and inflammation—used in combination with other pain-relievers	Drowsiness; dizziness; nausea; slurred speech	Confusion; reduced blood-cell counts; excitement; difficulty breathing; slow or irregular heart rate	Consult doctor before taking if you have liver disease. Dependence may result with extended use. Consult doctor before discontinuing this drug after extended use—withdrawal symptoms can occur, including agitation and seizures.
METHOCARBAMOL (Rx) **ROBAXIN** **DELAXIN** **ROBAXISAL***	Relieves muscle spasm and its pain	Dizziness; drowsiness; headache; loss of appetite; nausea	Allergic reactions, such as skin rash or itching	
METHYLPREDNIS-OLONE (Rx) **MEDROL**	All effects similar to CORTISOL			
NAPROXEN (Rx) **NAPROSYN**	All effects similar to FENOPROFEN			

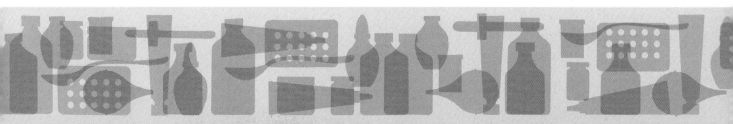

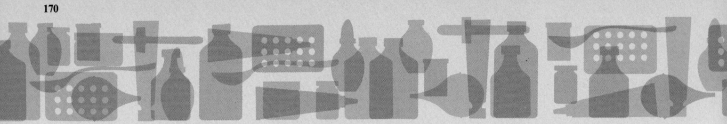

DRUG	Intended effect	Minor side effects	Serious side effects	Special cautions
ORPHENADRINE (Rx) **NORFLEX** **NORGESIC*** **NORGESIC FORTE***	Relieves muscle spasms and pain	Dry mouth; drowsiness; dizziness; nausea	Allergic reactions, such as skin rash or itching; fainting; mental confusion; rapid heart rate	Consult doctor before taking this drug if you have glaucoma, heart disease, ulcers, or obstruction of the urinary or intestinal tracts.
OXYCODONE (Rx) **PERCODAN*** **TYLOX*** **PERCOCET-5***	All effects similar to DIHYDROCODEINE BITARTRATE			
OXYPHENBUTAZONE (Rx) **TANDEARIL** **OXALID**	Relieves pain and inflammation, principally in arthritis	Nausea; vomiting; diarrhea	Stomach bleeding or ulcer; kidney damage; impaired vision; fluid retention; liver damage; reduced blood-cell counts	Consult doctor before taking if you have kidney or liver disease, or a history of stomach problems such as ulcers. Take with food or milk to decrease the likelihood or severity of stomach upset. Risk of ulcers is increased if this drug is taken with alcohol or other anti-inflammation drugs. Increased likelihood of bleeding if taken with warfarin sodium, a drug that thins the blood.
PENICILLAMINE (Rx) **CUPRIMINE**	Relieves rheumatoid-arthritis symptoms	Nausea; vomiting; altered taste; diarrhea	Allergic reactions, such as skin rash, itching and joint pain; reduced blood-cell counts; kidney damage; liver damage; muscle weakness; difficulty breathing; damage to eye nerves; extreme tiredness	Consult doctor before taking if you are pregnant—may cause deformities in the newborn. Consult doctor before taking if you have blood disorders or kidney, liver or respiratory disease. Avoid this drug if you have had allergic reactions to penicillin. Notify doctor of bloody or cloudy urine—signs of kidney damage. Effects interfered with by iron medications used to treat anemia—space doses at least 2 hours apart. Increased risk of blood-cell-count reductions if this drug is taken with phenylbutazone or oxyphenbutazone, drugs used to reduce inflammation and pain.
PENTAZOCINE (Rx) **TALWIN**	Relieves moderate to severe pain	Drowsiness; nausea; dizziness; constipation	Hallucinations; confusion; difficulty breathing	Consult doctor before taking if you have epilepsy or liver, kidney or heart disease, or recent head injury. Dependence can occur with extended use.
PHENYLBUTAZONE (Rx) **BUTAZOLIDIN**	All effects similar to OXYPHENBUTAZONE			
PHENYLTOLOXAMINE **PERCOGESIC***	Relieves anxiety that accompanies pain and inflammation; frequently used in combination with other pain relievers.	Drowsiness; dizziness; dry mouth; blurred vision; difficulty urinating	Rapid heart rate; hallucinations; confusion; delirium	Consult doctor before taking if you have glaucoma, heart disease, high blood pressure, or urinary or intestinal obstruction.
PREDNISOLONE (Rx) **DELTA-CORTEF** **STERANE** **ULACORT**	All effects similar to CORTISOL			

* Combination drug. Refer also to other active ingredients on label.

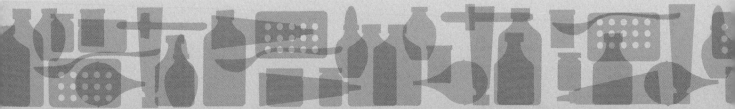

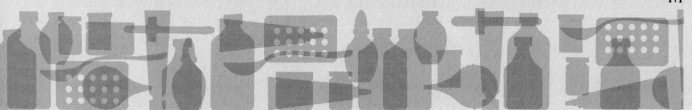

DRUG	Intended effect	Minor side effects	Serious side effects	Special cautions

PREDNISONE (Rx)
  DELTASONE
  ORASONE
  PARACORT
	All effects similar to CORTISOL			

PROBENECID (Rx)
  BENEMID
  COLBENEMID*
	Reduces uric-acid levels and prevents acute attacks of gout; helps control chronic gout	Nausea; vomiting; appetite loss; dizziness	Kidney stones; allergic reactions, such as skin rash, hives, wheezing, itching; reduced blood-cell counts	Consult doctor before taking if you have kidney stones, kidney disease, blood disorders or ulcers. Drink at least 10 glasses of water daily while taking this drug. Effects may be reduced by diuretics (drugs that cause fluid loss), aspirin and alcohol.

PROMETHAZINE (Rx)
  SYNALGOS*
  SYNALGOS-DC*
  MEPERGAN FORTIS*
	Relieves anxiety that may accompany pain; enhances pain-relieving action of other ingredients	Drowsiness; dizziness; dry mouth; blurred vision	Reduced blood-cell counts	Consult doctor before taking if you have blood disorders, liver disease or glaucoma.

PROPOXYPHENE (Rx)
  DARVON
  DOLENE
  DARVON-N
  DARVON COMPOUND-65*
	Relieves mild to moderate pain	Drowsiness; dizziness; nausea; constipation	Confusion; difficulty breathing; liver damage	Drug dependence may result from extended use.

SALSALATE (Rx)
  DISALCID
  ARCYLATE
	All effects similar to ASPIRIN			

SODIUM SALICYLATE **URACEL**	All effects similar to CHOLINE MAGNESIUM TRISALICYLATE			
SULFINPYRAZONE (Rx) **ANTURANE**	Prevents gout	Nausea; abdominal pain; vomiting	Peptic ulcer; skin rash; kidney stones; reduced blood-cell counts	Consult doctor before taking if you have ulcers, blood disorders, or allergies to phenylbutazone or oxyphenbutazone, anti-inflammation drugs. Take with food or milk to reduce stomach upset. Effects are reduced by diuretics (drugs that cause fluid loss), aspirin or alcohol. The effects of warfarin, a drug that thins the blood, may be increased by this drug. Drink at least 10 glasses of water daily while taking this drug.
SULINDAC (Rx) **CLINORIL**	All effects similar to FENOPROFEN			
TOLMETIN (Rx) **TOLECTIN**	All effects similar to FENOPROFEN			

TRIAMCINOLONE (Rx)
  ARISTOCORT
  KENACORT
	All effects similar to CORTISOL			

ZOMEPIRAC (Rx) **ZOMAX**	Relieves mild to severe pain and inflammation	Headache; nausea; dizziness; diarrhea; drowsiness	None	

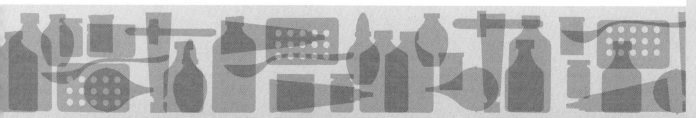

Bibliography

BOOKS

Adler, Philip, and George W. Northup, eds., *100 Years of Osteopathic Medicine*. Medical Communications, 1978.

Asimov, Isaac, *The Human Body: Its Structure and Operation*. New American Library, 1963.

Berland, Theodore, and Robert George Addison, *Living With Your Bad Back*. St. Martin's, 1972.

Brighton, Carl T., et al., eds., *Electrical Properties of Bone and Cartilage: Experimental Effects and Clinical Applications*. Grune & Stratton, 1979.

Cailliet, Rene:
Foot and Ankle Pain. F. A. Davis, 1968.
Low Back Pain Syndrome. F. A. Davis, 1968.

Calabro, John J., and John Wykert, *The Truth about Arthritis Care*. David McKay, 1971.

Corrigan, A. B., *Living With Arthritis*. Grosset & Dunlap, 1971.

Davis, Elwood Craig, and Gene A. Logan, *Biophysical Values of Muscular Activity with Implications for Research*. Wm. C. Brown, 1961.

DeVries, Herbert A., *Physiology of Exercise for Physical Education and Athletics*. Wm. C. Brown, 1980.

Engleman, Ephraim P., *The Arthritis Book*. Painter Hopkins, 1979.

Fahey, Thomas D., *What to Do about Athletic Injuries*. Butterick, 1979.

Finneson, Bernard E., and Arthur S. Freese, *Dr. Finneson on Low Back Pain*. G. P. Putnam's Sons, 1975.

Fixx, James F., *The Complete Book of Running*. Random House, 1977.

Fox, Edward L., *Sports Physiology*. W. B. Saunders, 1979.

Friedmann, Lawrence W., and Lawrence Galton, *Freedom from Backaches*. Simon and Schuster, 1973.

Fries, James F., *Arthritis: A Comprehensive Guide*. Addison-Wesley, 1979.

Gartland, John J., *Fundamentals of Orthopaedics*. W. B. Saunders, 1979.

Hall, Hamilton, *The Back Doctor: Ten Minutes a Day to Lifetime Relief for Your Aching Back*. McGraw-Hill, 1980.

Hanson, Isabel, *Outwitting Arthritis: People Talk about Coping With, Controlling & Conquering Arthritis*. Creative Arts, 1980.

Healey, Louis A., et al., *Beyond the Copper Bracelet: What You Should Know about Arthritis*. The Charles Press, 1977.

Helfet, Arthur J., and David M. Gruebel Lee, *Disorders of the Foot*. Lippincott, 1980.

Hubler, Richard G., *The Cristianis*. Little, Brown, 1966.

Inglis, Brian, *The Book of the Back*. Hearst Books, 1978.

Ishmael, William K., and Howard B. Shorbe, *Care of the Back*. Lippincott, 1976.

Jayson, Malcolm I. V., and Allan St. J. Dixon, *Understanding Arthritis and Rheumatism: A Complete Guide to the Problems and Treatment*. Random House, 1974.

Johnson, Lanny L., *Comprehensive Arthroscopic Examination of the Knee*. C. V. Mosby, 1977.

Kelsey, Jennifer L., et al., *Musculo-Skeletal Disorders: Their Frequency of Occurrence and Their Impact on the Population of the United States*. Neale Watson Academic Publications, 1978.

Key, James D., *The Week-End Athlete's Guide to Sports Medicine: Upper Body*. Anna Publishing, 1980.

Kraus, Hans, *Backache, Stress and Tension: Their Cause, Prevention and Treatment*. Simon & Schuster, 1965.

Lenihan, John, *Human Engineering: The Body Re-examined*. George Braziller, 1975.

Linde, Shirley Motter, *How to Beat a Bad Back: Hundreds of Things to Do to Achieve a Pain-Free Back*. Rawson, Wade, 1980.

Lorig, Kate, and James F. Fries, *The Arthritis Helpbook: What You Can Do for Your Arthritis*. Addison-Wesley, 1980.

McCarty, Daniel J., *Arthritis and Allied Conditions: A Textbook of Rheumatology*. Lea & Febiger, 1979.

MacCurdy, Edward, ed., *The Notebooks of Leonardo da Vinci*. George Braziller, 1958.

Mann, Roger A., ed., *DuVries' Surgery of the Foot*. C. V. Mosby, 1978.

Mirkin, Gabe, and Marshall Hoffman, *The Sportsmedicine Book*. Little, Brown, 1978.

Nourse, Alan E., *Fractures, Dislocations, and Sprains*. Franklin Watts, 1978.

Perkins, Faith, *My Fight with Arthritis*. Random House, 1964.

The Rand McNally Atlas of the Body and Mind. Rand McNally with Mitchell Beazley, 1976.

Root, Leon, and Thomas Kiernan, *Oh, My Aching Back: A Doctor's Guide to Your Back Pain and How to Control It*. David McKay, 1973.

Rosse, Cornelius, and D. Kay Clawson, *The Musculoskeletal System in Health and Disease*. Harper & Row, 1980.

Samachson, Joseph, *The Armor within Us: The Story of Bone*. Rand McNally, 1966.

Schneider, Myles J., and Mark D. Sussman,

How to Doctor Your Feet without the Doctor. Running Times, 1980.

Singer, Sam, and Henry R. Hilgard, *The Biology of People*. W. H. Freeman, 1978.

PERIODICALS

Brighton, Carl T., et al., "A Multicenter Study of the Treatment of Non-Union with Constant Direct Current." *The Journal of Bone and Joint Surgery*, Vol. 63-A, No. 1, January 1981.

Brody, David M., "Running Injuries." *Clinical Symposia*, Vol. 32, No. 4, 1980.

"Chiropractors: Healers or Quacks? Part 1: The 80-Year War with Science." *Consumer Reports*, September 1975.

"Chiropractors: Healers or Quacks? Part 2: How Chiropractors Can Help—or Harm." *Consumer Reports*, October 1975.

Farah, Adelaide P., "Meet Your Feet." *Family Health*, July 1975.

Fettner, Ann G., "Sir John Charnley: Arthritis Pioneer." *The National Arthritis News*, Vol. 2, No. 2, Spring 1981.

Journal of the American Podiatry Association, Vol. 68, No. 4, April 1978.

"Muscles, Bones, and Numbers." *Mosaic*, November/December 1976.

Poehling, Gary G., "Arthroscopy." *Physical Therapy*, Vol. 60, No. 12, December 1980.

Salter, Robert B., "Etiology, Pathogenesis and Possible Prevention of Congenital Dislocation of the Hip." *The Canadian Medical Association Journal*, Vol. 98, No. 20, May 18, 1968.

Treaster, Joseph B., "Ballet: The Agony behind the Ecstasy." *Family Health*, October 1978.

OTHER PUBLICATIONS

"Chiropractic: State of the Art." American Chiropractic Association, May 1981.

Pogoloff, Christina, and Ruth Silverstone, "A Really Big Shoe—a Summary." Consumer Survival Kit, Maryland Center for Public Broadcasting, 1975.

Picture credits

The sources for the illustrations that appear in this book are listed below. Credits for the illustrations from left to right are separated by semicolons, from top to bottom by dashes.

Cover: Fil Hunter. 7: Fil Hunter. 9: Keystone Press Agency, London. 11: Herbert Migdoll, courtesy Joffrey Ballet. 12: Arthur Elgort. 13: Herbert Migdoll, courtesy Joffrey Ballet. 15: William Campbell; Victor Englebert from Photo Researchers. 17-19: Drawings by Trudy Nicholson. 22-25: Linda Bartlett. 26: The Children's Hospital of Philadelphia—Linda Bartlett. 27-35: Linda Bartlett. 37: Robert Frerck. 39: Guido Sansoni, courtesy Biblioteca Medicea-Laurenziana, Florence. 41: Walter Hilmers Jr. from HJ Commercial Art. 43-45: Robert Frerck. 48, 49: Drawings by Trudy Nicholson. 51: Walter Hilmers Jr. from HJ Commercial Art. 55-57: Richard Anderson. 59: Still National Osteopathic Museum. 60-65: Frederic F. Bigio from B-C Graphics. 67: Henry Groskinsky. 69: Drawings by Jane Hurd, courtesy Dr. Rene Cailliet from *Foot and Ankle Pain,* F. A. Davis Publishing, 1974. 70, 71: Walter Hilmers Jr. from HJ Commercial Art. 73: Drawing by Karen Karlsson. 75: Drawings by Joan McGurren. 77: John Senzer, courtesy The Langer Group. 78, 79: John Senzer. 81: Scholl, Inc. 83: John Zimmerman. 84: Drawing by Trudy Nicholson. 86: McDavid Knee Guard, Inc. 89: Drawing by Trudy Nicholson. 90, 94: Walter Hilmers Jr. from HJ Commercial Art. 96: John Senzer. 97: Walter Hilmers Jr. From HJ Commercial Art. 98, 99: John Senzer. 100, 101: John Senzer (2)—Walter Hilmers Jr. from HJ Commercial Art. 102-107: John Senzer. 109: © Howard Sochurek, 1981. 111: Drawings by Joan McGurren. 112: Mary Evans Picture Library, London. 114-116: Zoological Society of San Diego. 119: Reprinted from *The Journal of Bone and Joint Surgery,* Vols. 44-A, No. 7 & 50-A, No. 4 (1962/68), courtesy F. W. Rhinelander, M.D., Orthopaedic Hospital-USC, U.S.P.H.S. Research Grant (No. AM 27625). 121: © 1980 Burt Glinn from Magnum. 122: Courtesy ZIMMER/ProClinica. 123: Courtesy ZIMMER/ProClinica—© 1980 Burt Glinn from Magnum. 125: Joe McNally for DISCOVER. 127: Enrico Ferorelli, courtesy Spain Rehabilitation Center, University of Alabama in Birmingham. 129, 130: Walter Hilmers Jr. from HJ Commercial Art. 132, 133: Enrico Ferorelli, courtesy Spain Rehabilitation Center, University of Alabama in Birmingham. 134: S. Gay and L. Balleisen, ''Components of the Lesion and Regression,'' from *Atherosclerosis—Is It Reversible?* Ed. by G. Schettler, E. Stange, R. W. Wissler, Springer Verlag, Berlin-Heidelberg-New York, 1972. 135: S. Gay and E. G. Miller, *Collagen in the Physiology and Pathology of Connective Tissue.* Gustav Fischer, Stuttgart-New York, 1978. 137: Erich Lessing, courtesy Kunsthistorisches Museum, Vienna.

140: David Strick for DISCOVER. 142, 143: David Lees, Florence. 144: Fil Hunter, insert, Orthopedic Products/3M. 146-159: Enrico Ferorelli. 166-171: Frederic F. Bigio from B-C Graphics.

Acknowledgments

The index for this book was prepared by B. L. Klein. For their help in the preparation of this volume, the editors wish to thank the following: P. F. Adams, National Center for Health Statistics, Hyattsville, Md.; Dr. J. L. Albrigo, National Hospital for Orthopaedics and Rehabilitation, Arlington, Va.; M. Andrews, International Shrine Headquarters, Tampa, Fla.; M. Baker, San Diego Wild Animal Park, Escondido, Calif.; Dr. J. C. Bennett, University of Alabama, Birmingham; K. Bilson, University of Alabama, Birmingham; Dr. G. P. Bogumill, Georgetown University Hospital, Washington, D.C.; K. Braun, Sports Medicine Center, Chevy Chase, Md.; Dr. C. T. Brighton, University of Pennsylvania School of Medicine, Philadelphia; Dr. D. Brody, Sports Medicine Center, Chevy Chase, Md.; L. Buttell, American Podiatry Association, Washington, D.C.; A. C. Collier, University of Alabama Hospitals, Birmingham; H. Coviello, Arlington, Tenn.; Dr. M. K. Dalinka, University of Pennsylvania Hospital, Philadelphia; H. DeLuca, University of Wisconsin, Madison; B. Denman, Memphis, Tenn.; Dr. J. Doherty, New York City; Dr. M. L. Ecker, Children's Hospital of Philadelphia, Pa.; Dr. R. D. Ellis, Children's Hospital of Philadelphia, Pa.; J. Emond, The Langer Group, Deer Park, N.Y.; P. S. Esterson, National Hospital for Orthopaedics and Rehabilitation, Arlington, Va.; A. Fettner, Arthritis Foundation, Atlanta, Ga.; P. Couillard Freese, St. Paul, Minn.; Dr. S. Gay, University Medical Center, Birmingham, Ala.; G. S. George, University of Southwestern Louisiana, Lafayette; Dr. N. L. Gerber, National Institutes of Health, Bethesda, Md.; Dr. D. Gershuni, La Jolla, Calif.; Dr. H. Hall, Canadian Back Education Units, Toronto, Ont.; R. Hollander, National Center for Health Statistics, Hyattsville, Md.; Dr. J. M. Hunter, Hand Rehabilitation Center, Philadelphia, Pa.; Dr. S. H. Jaeger, Hand Rehabilitation Center, Philadelphia, Pa.; J. N. Kalonturos, Owens Chiropractic Clinic, Waldorf, Md.; N. Klombers, American Podiatry Association, Washington, D.C.; Dr. W. Koopman, University of Alabama, Birmingham; C. E. Krausz, Cheltenham, Pa.; Dr. S. Lavine, Washington, D.C.; J. LeFace, The Langer Group, Deer Park, N.Y.; L. Lombardo, Children's Hospital of Philadelphia, Pa.; J. D. Lynn, University of Alabama, Birmingham; P. Mathon, Arthritis Foundation, Atlanta, Ga.; G. Matthews, Braintree, Mass.; Dr. J. G. Matthews II, Naval Medical Research Institute, Bethesda, Md.; R. F. McDavid III, Clarendon Hills, Ill.; Dr. J. Miller, University of Illinois, Chicago; Dr. M. L. Miller, Rockville, Md.; M. Molnar, New York City Ballet, New York City; J. P. Mustone, The Exercise Exchange, New York City; O. Myers, American Red Cross, Washington, D.C.; A. H. Navarro, Johns Hopkins University School of Medicine, Baltimore, Md.; Dr. L. Ng, National Institute on Drug Abuse, Washington, D.C.; D. B. Owens, Owens Chiropractic Clinic, Waldorf, Md.; J. Palmer, Eli Lilly and Company, Indianapolis, Ind.; J. W. Parker, University of Alabama, Birmingham; B. A. Patrissi, Arthritis Foundation, Washington, D.C.; Dr. T. J. Pekin, Jr., Georgetown University Medical Center, Washington, D.C.; W. Penney, Children's Hospital of Philadelphia, Pa.; Dr. R. B. Pitkow, Children's Hospital of Philadelphia, Pa.; W. E. Plunkett, National Arthritis Advisory Board, Bethesda, Md.; M. Polcahninoff, The Langer Group, Deer Park, N.Y.; P. B. Porter, University of Alabama, Birmingham; Mr. and Mrs. E. Purinton, Linwood, N.J.; Dr. F. W. Rhinelander, University of Southern California School of Medicine, Los Angeles; J. Romero, Sports Medicine Center, Chevy Chase, Md.; R. Scamardi, Children's Hospital of Philadelphia, Pa.; Dr. A. B. Schultz, University of Illinois, Chicago; Dr. R. O. Schuster, Merritt Island, Fla.; D. Simons, National Hospital for Orthopaedics and Rehabilitation, Arlington, Va.; Dr. M. B. Stevens, Johns Hopkins University School of Medicine, Baltimore, Md.; J. Sutton, Johns Hopkins University School of Medicine, Baltimore, Md.; M. A. Taylor, Children's Hospital of Philadelphia, Pa.; Dr. J. S. Torg, University of Pennsylvania, Philadelphia; J. J. Vegso, University of Pennsylvania, Philadelphia; Dr. D. Wallace, Los Angeles; Dr. J. F. Waller, New York City; D. Warwick, University of Illinois, Chicago; Dr. H. G. Watts, Children's Hospital of Philadelphia, Pa.; J. Wernick, The Langer Group, Deer Park, N.Y.; Dr. S. Wiesel, George Washington University Medical Center, Washington, D.C.; Dr. R. Windsor, Children's Hospital of Philadelphia, Pa.; B. Woodward, Scottsdale, Ariz.; J. L. Wright, Jr., University of Alabama Hospitals, Birmingham; M. Yaslow, Pro Clinica, New York City; J. M. Yonts, American Osteopathic Association, Chicago.

Index